Adult and Paediatric ALS

Self-assessment in Resuscitation

Adult and Paediatric ALS

Self-assessment in Resuscitation

Charles D. Deakin MA MD FRCP FRCA FERC FFICM

Honorary Professor of Resuscitation and Prehospital Emergency Medicine, University of Southampton, UK
Consultant in Cardiac Anaesthesia and Intensive Care, University Hospital Southampton, UK
Executive Committee, Resuscitation Council (UK)
Immediate Past Chair, Advanced Life Support Committee, European Resuscitation Council
Immediate Past Co-Chair, Advanced Life Support Committee, International Liaison Committee on Resuscitation

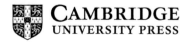

CAMBRIDGE UNIVERSITY PRESS
Cambridge, New York, Melbourne, Madrid, Cape Town,
Singapore, São Paulo, Delhi, Mexico City

Cambridge University Press
The Edinburgh Building, Cambridge CB2 8RU, UK

Published in the United States of America by
Cambridge University Press, New York

www.cambridge.org
Information on this title: www.cambridge.org/
9781107616301

First published 2012

Printed in the United Kingdom at the
MPG Books Group

*A catalogue record for this publication is available from the
British Library*

Library of Congress Cataloguing in Publication data
Deakin, Charles D.
Adult and paediatric ALS : self-assessment in resuscitation /
Charles D. Deakin.
  p.   ;   cm.
Adult and paediatric advanced life support
Includes index.
ISBN 978-1-107-61630-1 (pbk.)
I. Title.   II. Title: Adult and paediatric advanced life support.
[DNLM: 1. Resuscitation – Examination Questions.   2. Life
Support Care – Examination Questions. WA 18.2]
616.1′025076 – dc23   2011049190

ISBN 978-1-107-61630-1 Paperback

Contents

Dedication

To my daughter, Maddie, with apologies for her encounter with sevoflurane!
To my parents, Mary and David
To all my friends at the Resuscitation Council (UK)

Preface

Basic and advanced life support courses are under-taken by most NHS clinical staff and resuscitation is a mandatory area of knowledge. Those preparing for a resuscitation course, or those wishing to maintain and update their knowledge, may enjoy an alternative to course manuals and resuscitation texts in the form of these short test papers in resuscitation.

The book covers the entire basic and advanced life support syllabus for both adult and paediatric resuscitation, each section comprising 20 multiple choice questions, five photographic questions, five diagnostic questions and five short answers. This book is intended for all those taking advanced life support courses and those taking higher medical examinations that include a resuscitation component, so covers core knowledge needed by all specialist trainees and consultants in acute medical specialities.

Abbreviations

AC	Alternating current	IO	Intraosseous
ACE	Angiotensin-converting enzyme	IV	Intravenous
AED	Automatic external defibrillator	LMA	Laryngeal mask airway
AICD	Automatic implantable cardioverter–defibrillator	LUCAS	Lund University Cardiac Assist System
		NICE	National Institute for Clinical Excellence
AIDS	Aquired immunodeficiency syndrome	$Paco_2$	Arterial partial pressure of carbon dioxide
ALS	Advanced life support		
BLS	Basic life support	PEA	Pulseless electrical activity
CNS	Central nervous system	Pao_2	Arterial partial pressure of oxygen
CPR	Cardiopulmonary resuscitation	PEEP	Positive end-expiratory pressure
CVC	Central venous catheter	Pco_2	Partial pressure carbon dioxide
CVP	Central venous pressure	Po_2	Partial pressure oxygen
CXR	Chest radiograph	Sao_2	Arterial haemoglobin oxygen saturation
DC	Direct current	SC	Subcutaneous
ECG	Electrocardiography	Spo_2	Arterial haemoglobin oxygen saturation measured non-invasively by pulse oximetry
GTN	Glyceryl trinitrate (nitroglycerin)		
HIV	Human immunodeficiency virus		
IABP	Intra-aortic balloon pump	VF	Ventricular fibrillation
ICD	Internal cardioverter device	VT	Ventricular tachycardia
IM	Intramuscular	TRALI	Transfusion-related acute lung injury
IN	Intranasal		

Multiple choice questions

Question 1

A 15:2 compression:ventilation ratio is recommended for resuscitation of:

a. adults, if the rescuer is trained
b. adults, if the rescuer is untrained
c. children less than 8 years old, if the rescuer is untrained
d. children less than 8 years old, if the rescuer is trained
e. adult drowning victims.

Question 2

Which of the following are correct doses for paediatric cardiac arrest?

a. atropine 10 μg/kg
b. adrenaline (epinephrine) 10 μg/kg
c. amiodarone 10 μg/kg
d. defibrillation (monophasic defibrillator) 4 J/kg
e. defibrillation (biphasic defibrillator) 2 J/kg.

Question 3

Which of the following statements are correct?

a. in an adult male (70–80 kg), the endotracheal tube should be 26 cm length at the lips
b. a size 4 laryngeal mask airway (LMA) is suitable for most adults
c. a size 9.0 mm nasopharyngeal airway is suitable for most adults
d. the size of an endotracheal tube, e.g. 7.0 mm, refers to its external diameter
e. a size 2 or 3 oropharyngeal airway is generally suitable for an 8-year-old patient.

Question 4

Which of the following drugs cause pupillary dilation?

a. atropine
b. adrenaline
c. amiodarone
d. lignocaine
e. sodium bicarbonate.

Question 5

With regard to cardiac arrest:

a. the commonest cause in adults is ischaemic heart disease
b. home defibrillators for high-risk patients double survival rates
c. paediatric cardiac arrest is usually due to a final common pathway causing hypoxaemia
d. bystander cardiopulmonary resuscitation (CPR) doubles the survival rate
e. sudden cardiac death accounts for about 15% of all deaths in Western countries.

Question 6

With regard to amiodarone:

a. hypotension results from histamine release
b. should be administered if the patient remains in VF after the second shock
c. the initial adult dose is 300 mg IV
d. may cause optic neuritis with prolonged use
e. precipitates with adrenaline.

Question 7

In diagnosing heat stroke in a pyrexial patient, the following differential diagnoses should be considered:

a. neuroleptic malignant syndrome
b. phaeochromocytoma
c. hypothyroidism
d. anaphylaxis
e. CNS infection.

Question 8

Noradrenaline (norepinephrine):

a. is principally an α-agonist
b. has some β-agonist action
c. may cause a reflex bradycardia
d. is synthesized primarily in the adrenal cortex
e. is broken down into various metabolites that include adrenaline.

Question 9

ECG changes of hypothermia include:

a. shortened PR interval
b. flattened T wave
c. J wave
d. movement artefact from shivering
e. VF.

Question 10

Suitable positions for self-adhesive pad placement for defibrillation of VF include:

a. biaxillary
b. anterior (right sternal edge) and left axilla
c. anterior (left sternal edge) and left axilla
d. anterior (left sternal edge) and posterior
e. anterior (right sternal edge) and posterior.

Question 11

The following drugs cause hypotension through histamine release:

a. atracurium
b. fentanyl
c. morphine
d. amitriptyline
e. midazolam.

Question 12

With regard to O_2:

a. the concentration in exhaled breath is 18%
b. 30% O_2 doubles the rate of combustion
c. in most tissues of the body, the response to hypoxia is vasodilatation
d. in the lungs, the response to hypoxia is vasoconstriction
e. hyperventilation increases O_2 uptake.

Question 13

Pulse oximetry:

a. the presence of carbon monoxide in the blood (COHb) results in an overestimation of oxygen saturation of haemoglobin (Sao_2)
b. the presence of methaemoglobin in the blood (MetHb) results in an overestimation of Sao_2
c. fetal Hb results in an overestimation of Sao_2
d. a poor pulse oximetry trace may result in an underestimation of Sao_2
e. diathermy may interfere with waveform detection.

Question 14

With regard to capnography:

a. normal range is approximately 4.5–6.0 kPa
b. absence of endotracheal end-tidal CO_2 during a cardiac arrest is diagnostic of oesophageal intubation
c. end-tidal CO_2 that does not rise above 1.4 kPa (10 mmHg) during a resuscitation attempt is associated with a poor prognosis
d. cooling increases end-tidal CO_2
e. $Paco_2$ is equal to end-tidal CO_2.

Question 15

With regard to severe local anaesthetic toxicity associated with cardiovascular collapse:

a. lignocaine is the commonest local anaesthetic implicated in this condition
b. may benefit from administration of Intralipid 20%
c. propofol (an intralipid emulsion) is a suitable alternative to Intralipid
d. the maximum recommended safe dose of bupivacaine is 2 mg/kg IV
e. survival is uncommon.

Question 16

How should chest compressions be performed on an infant?

a. with the heel of one hand and the other hand on top of the first
b. with the heel of one hand only
c. with 4 fingers of one hand
d. with 2 fingers of one hand
e. with the thumb of one hand.

Question 17

If an AED is available, but adult self-adhesive pads are available, how should you manage a 5-year-old child in cardiac arrest with a shockable rhythm?

a. AED use is unnecessary as shockable rhythms are rare in this age group
b. use the AED, but apply only one of the pads
c. use the AED with adult pads
d. perform CPR, but do not use the AED
e. use the AED for a single shock only.

Question 18

With regard to drug doses:

a. 1 ml 1:1000 adrenaline $=$ 1 mg adrenaline
b. 10 ml 0.25% bupivacaine $=$ 25 mg bupivacaine
c. 100 µg (mcg) adrenaline $=$ 1 ml 1:10 000 adrenaline
d. 1 mg IV adrenaline has the same efficacy as ~2 mg IO (intraosseous) adrenaline
e. 10 ml 50% dextrose $=$ 100 ml 5% dextrose.

Question 19

A pacemaker programmed to:

a. AOO paces and senses the atrium only
b. VVI paces and senses the atrium only
c. DDD paces and senses both the atrium and ventricle
d. DDDR has the capability to defibrillate
e. DDD may be inhibited by diathermy current.

Question 20

With regard to haemorrhage:

a. circulating blood volume in an adult is approximately 4% of body mass
b. patients who have an impaired level of consciousness due to blood loss have generally lost at least 40% of their circulating blood volume
c. β-blockers may mask the early signs of hypovolaemic shock
d. the management of catastrophic haemorrhage should take priority over airway management
e. venous bleeding is generally less serious than arterial bleeding.

Photograph questions

Question 1

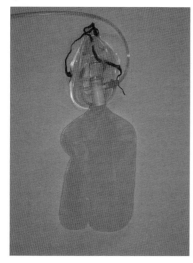

a. What is this?
b. What is the function of the reservoir?
c. What O_2 flow rate delivers 100% O_2 to the patient?

Question 2

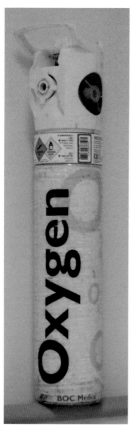

a. What is the percentage of O_2 in the atmosphere?
b. What volume of gas is discharged from this CD size cylinder?
c. Why does the cylinder become cold during use?

Question 3

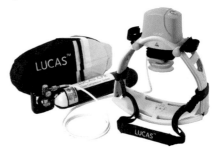

a. What is this?
b. How is this device powered?
c. What hazards may be associated with its use during defibrillation?

Question 4

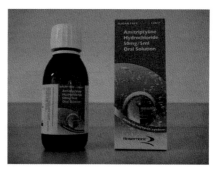

a. What class of medication is this solution?
b. What ECG changes does it cause when taken as an overdose?
c. How is this overdose treated?

Question 5

This device can be placed over implanted pacemakers or cardioverter–defibrillators.

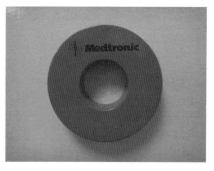

a. What is it?
b. What is its effect on an implantable pacemaker?
c. What is its effect on an automated implantable cardioverter–defibrillator (AICD)?

Diagnostic questions

Question 1

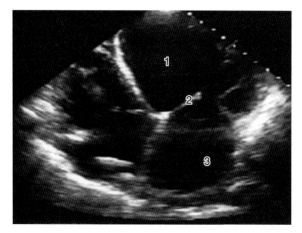

a. What is this image?
b. Name structures 1–3.

Question 2

This is a paced ECG. What mode is the pacemaker set to?

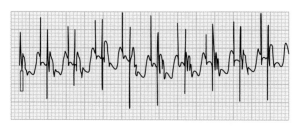

Question 3

The following results have been obtained:

Na^+	135 mmol/l
K^+	7.2 mmol/l
urea	33.4 mmol/l
creatinine	488 mmol/l
glucose	18.9 mmol/l

a. What is the most immediate priority in this patient?
b. Which organ system is failing?
c. What is the likely cause of this failure?

Question 4

An arterial blood gas sample (on air) is taken from an unresponsive patient, with the following results:

pH	7.21
Pao_2	11.0 kPa
$Paco_2$	8.8 kPa
HCO_3^-	15 mmol/l

a. What metabolic derangement is seen in this blood gas?
b. Name three likely causes.

Question 5

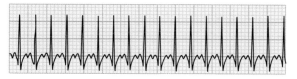

a. What rhythm does this ECG show?
b. What non-pharmacological methods may be used to terminate the arrhythmia?
c. What pharmacological methods may be used to terminate the arrhythmia?

Short answer questions

Question 1

Draw the algorithm for paediatric ALS.

Question 2

Explain why dextrose-containing solutions are contraindicated as resuscitation fluids.

Question 3

How quickly does manual external chest compression fatigue? How often should rescuers change?

Question 4

What are the risks of performing a needle pericardiocentesis? How may these risks be minimized?

Question 5

Draw a cross-section of the heart to show the right atrium and ventricle, left atrium and ventricle and pulmonary artery and aorta. Label each with normal values for O_2 saturation (on air).

MCQ answers

Answer 1

a. **False.** 30:2 is recommended in adults, irrespective of whether the rescuer is trained or untrained.
b. **False.**
c. **False.** 30:2 is recommended in children if the rescuer is untrained.
d. **False.** Trained rescuers should use 15:2.
e. **True.**

Answer 2

a. **False.** Atropine is not recommended for routine use. When it is given, the correct dose is 20 µg/kg.
b. **True.** 100 µg/kg should be considered in children with cardiac arrest associated with severe vasodilation, e.g. sepsis.
c. **False.** Amiodarone 5 mg/kg for both the first and, if given, the second dose.
d. **True.**
e. **False.** The recommended energy level for biphasic defibrillators is also 4 J/kg for all shocks.

Answer 3

a. **False.** For a 70–80 kg adult, the endotracheal tube should be 22–24 cm at the lips.
b. **True.**
c. **False.** A size 6.0–7.0 mm airway is adequate for most adults.
d. **False.** The size refers to the internal diameter.
e. **True.**

Answer 4

a. **True.**
b. **True.**
c. **False.**
d. **False.**
e. **False.**

Answer 5

a. **True.** Among adults, ischaemic heart disease is the predominant cause of arrest, with 30% of people at autopsy showing signs of recent myocardial infarction.
b. **False.** Home defibrillators have not been shown to improve outcome from cardiac arrest.
c. **True.**

d. **True.**
e. **False.** 30%.

Answer 6

a. **False.** Hypotension is thought to be caused by the solvent in which amiodarone is dissolved.
b. **False.** Amiodarone is indicated immediately after the third shock.
c. **True.**
d. **True.**
e. **Frue.**

Answer 7

a. **True.**
b. **True.**
c. **False.** Hyperthyroidism.
d. **False.**
e. **True.**

Answer 8

a. **True.**
b. **True.**
c. **True.**
d. **False.** Is synthesized primarily in the adrenal medulla.
e. **True.**

Answer 9

a. **False.** Prolonged PR interval.
b. **True.**
c. **True.**
d. **True.**
e. **True.** Asystole and VF may begin spontaneously at core temperatures below 25–28°C.

Answer 10

a. **True.**
b. **True.**
c. **False.**
d. **True.**
e. **True.**

Answer 11

a. **True.**
b. **False.**
c. **True.**
d. **False.**
e. **False.**

Answer 12

a. **False.** 15%.
b. **False.** 24% O_2 doubles the rate of combustion. 30% increases the rate 10-fold.
c. **True.**
d. **True.** This is known as hypoxic pulmonary vasoconstriction.
e. **False.**

Answer 13

a. **True.** At 660 nm (used by the pulse oximeter), COHb absorbs light in a similar manner to HbO_2.
b. **False.** At 660 nm, MetHb has similar absorption to reduced Hb. Sao_2 decreases with increasing MetHb levels, towards a Sao_2 of 85%. Below 85%, the presence of MetHb will, therefore, result in an increase in Sao_2 towards 85%.
c. **False.** Fetal Hb has no significant effect on pulse oximetry values.
d. **True.**
e. **True.**

Answer 14

a. **True.**
b. **False.** Also occurs with no cardiac output.
c. **False.** A threshold value of 10 mmHg (1.4 kPa) as a prognosticator for irreversible death in out-of-hospital cardiac arrest has been demonstrated (Levine RL *et al. N Engl J Med*, 1995;337:301–306; Cantineau JP *et al. Crit Care Med*, 1996;24:791–796).
d. **False.** Cooling reduces metabolic rate and cardiac output, subsequently reducing end-tidal CO_2.
e. **False.** When ventilation and perfusion are equal, $Paco_2$ is equal to end-tidal CO_2. In practice, however, there is always a degree of shunting within the lungs, resulting in less-efficient gas transfer. In conditions such as cardiac arrest, chronic obstructive pulmonary disease or adult respiratory distress syndrome, an even greater ventilation/perfusion abnormality occurs and high CO_2 gradients result.

Answer 15

a. **False.** Bupivacaine.
b. **True.** Some animal studies and human case reports suggest that Intralipid may be of benefit in these patients (Soar J *et al. Resuscitation*, 2010;81:1400–1433).

c. **False.** Propofol is dissolved in Intralipid, but at inadequate dose to be in the therapeutic range.
d. **True.**
e. **True.** Bupivacaine is thought to bind strongly to myocardial tissue and its effects are difficult to reverse.

Answer 16

a. **False.**
b. **False.**
c. **False.**
d. **True.**
e. **False.**

Answer 17

a. **False.**
b. **False.**
c. **True.**
d. **False.**
e. **False.**

Answer 18

a. **True.**
b. **True.** A 1% solution contains 10 mg/ml.
c. **True.**
d. **False.** IV and IO routes have the same bioavailability and, therefore, efficacy.
e. **True.**

Answer 19

a. **False.** AOO paces the atrium only and is not inhibited by atrial or ventricular activity.
b. **False.** VVI paces the ventricle and is inhibited by ventricular activity.
c. **True.**
d. **False.** 'R' means that the device is rate responsive and can vary its rate.
e. **True.** Electrical activity from diathermy devices can be sensed by pacemakers, which then mistakenly inhibit output.

Answer 20

a. **False.** 7%.
b. **True.**
c. **True.** Tachycardia may be masked by β-blockers.
d. **True.** The traditional ABC approach has been superseded by cABC, where the initial priority is to stop any torrential haemorrhage (e.g. from limb amputation) prior to moving on to ABC.
e. **False.**

Photograph answers

Answer 1

a. Oxygen rebreathing mask.

b. The reservoir fills with O_2 to provide additional O_2 to that delivered when the patient inhales.

c. A rate of 15 l/min O_2 results in the patient inhaling approximately 85–90% O_2; 100% O_2 is only possible with sealed systems.

Answer 2

a. 21%.

b. This is a CD size O_2 cylinder, which stores 460 litres.

c. Pressure of a gas (P) is related to its volume (V), given by the equation $P/V = k$, where k is a constant. Also, P is proportional to the absolute temperature (T; measured in Kelvin) of the gas. Therefore, as gas escapes from a pressurized cylinder (137 bar when full), the pressure falls and the gas remaining in the cylinder expands. This fall in pressure results in a proportional temperature decrease.

Answer 3

a. Lund University Cardiac Assist System (LUCAS) (Deakin CD *et al. Resuscitation*, 2010;81:1305–1352).

b. The device is powered by compressed O_2 at >100 l/min. Later devices (LUCAS2) are powered by battery.

c. The exhaust O_2 gas discharged from the device results in high ambient O_2 concentrations, particularly in confined spaces. High ambient O_2 concentrations are a risk for fire or explosion.

Answer 4

a. Tricyclic antidepressant.

b. Prolonged QTc, widened QRS complex, ventricular fibrillation (VF).

c. In patients with a metabolic acidosis, sodium bicarbonate (IV) is recommended. The postulated mechanism of action is two-fold:
   - tricyclics are protein bound but less so in acidic conditions; reversing the acidosis increases protein binding and decreases bioavailability of the drug
   - sodium load may help to reverse the sodium channel blocking effects of the tricyclic drug
   - treatment is otherwise supportive.

Answer 5

a. Ring magnet.

b. The magnet inhibits sensing by the pacemaker, converting to a fixed output mode (e.g. AOO) at a preset rate (usually 50/min).

c. The magnet will have the same effect on the pacing function of an AICD as for an implantable pacemaker (b). It will also inhibit the defibrillation function of the device.

Diagnostic answers

Answer 1

a. Structures are:

(1) left ventricle
(2) mitral valve
(3) left atrium.

The figure shows the orientation:

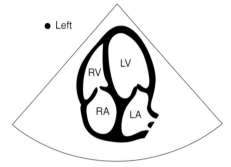

Answer 2

DDD. Both atrial (red arrows) and ventricular (blue arrows) pacing spikes can be seen.

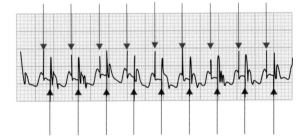

Answer 3

a. The immediate priority in this patient is the treatment of hyperkalaemia (normal range 3.5–5.0 mmol/l).
b. The urea (normal range 3.0–7.0 mmol/l) and creatinine (normal range 50–118 mmol/l) are both significantly elevated, suggesting renal failure; the likely cause of this is hyperkalaemia.
c. The high glucose level (normal range 3.0–7.0 mmol/l) is suggestive of diabetes, a common cause of chronic renal failure.

Answer 4

a. Acute respiratory acidosis.
b. Respiratory depression, respiratory failure, airway obstruction, hypoventilation from a low minute volume of any cause.

Answer 5

a. Supraventricular tachycardia (with a rate approximately 300/min).
b. Carotid sinus massage, sucking ice, cold flannel over the face.
c. Adenosine 3–6 mg IV; verapamil 2.5–5 mg IV boluses are an alternative if adenosine is not available.

Short answers

Answer 1

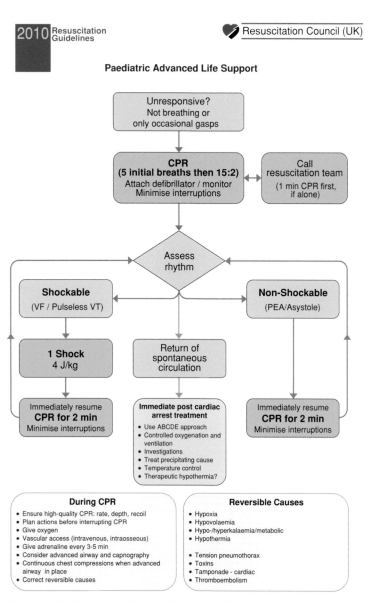

Reproduced with permission from the Resuscitation Council (UK).

Answer 2

Solutions containing dextrose (sugar) are contraindicated in resuscitation because:

- hyperglycaemia may exacerbate cellular ischaemic damage; there is some evidence that hyperglycaemia caused by dextrose-containing fluids given during resuscitation may worsen outcome

- dextrose is rapidly metabolized to leave free water, which remains in the intravascular space for a very short period before entering the extravascular space; consequently its volume-expanding effects are very limited, 1000 ml 5% dextrose will expand the intravascular space by just 67 ml.

Answer 3

Manual external chest compression fatigues after 1 min, although rescuers do not perceive that they are suffering fatigue until approximately 3 min of performing chest compressions. Ideally, the individual performing chest compression should change after no more than 2 min (Javier OF, *et al. Resuscitation*, 1988;37:149–152).

Answer 4

Acute risks of needle pericardiocentesis include:

- myocardial puncture
- coronary artery puncture
- myocardial infarction
- needle-induced arrhythmias
- pneumopericardium
- pneumothorax
- accidental puncture of the liver, stomach or lung.

Risks can be minimized by using transthoracic echo or fluoroscopy to ensure correct placement of the needle. Use of an ECG injury potential when the needle penetrates the myocardium is no longer a recommended technique.

Answer 5

Normal O_2 saturations (on air):

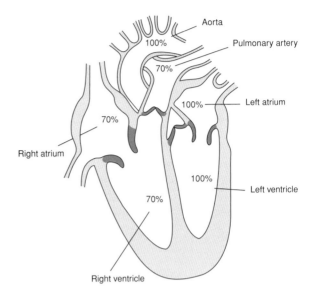

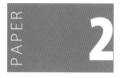
Multiple choice questions

Question 1

With regard to potassium metabolism:

a. the normal potassium level is 3.0–5.5 mmol/l
b. hyperkalaemia is defined as $K^+ > 5.5$ mmol/l
c. hyperkalaemia is exacerbated by alkalosis
d. hyperkalaemia is common with acute renal failure
e. hyperkalaemia may be caused by haemolysis of a blood sample.

Question 2

Positive pressure ventilation causes:

a. decreased cardiac output
b. increased venous return
c. increased renal blood flow
d. raised intracerebral pressure
e. respiratory muscle atrophy.

Question 3

Hard collars for cervical spine immobilization:

a. are contraindicated in patients with base of skull fracture
b. may cause pressure sores
c. may decrease cerebral perfusion pressure
d. should be fitted after the airway has been secured
e. can be loosened if a patient's head is stabilized on a spinal board between head blocks.

Question 4

A child's weight (kg) can be estimated from the following equation:

a. Weight $= 2(\text{age} + 4)$
b. Weight $= (\text{age}/4) + 4$
c. Weight $= 7(\text{age})/3$
d. Weight $= 3(\text{age} - 4)$
e. Weight $= 3(\text{age}) + 7$.

Question 5

In the management of burns:

a. Body surface area calculations exclude erythematous areas
b. the whole hand represents 1% body surface area
c. children have proportionately larger heads than adults
d. fluid requirements are calculated from the time of the burn occurring, not the time treatment starts
e. airway swelling from respiratory tract burns is at its worst 2–4 h after the burn has occurred.

Question 6

Intraosseous access:

a. should be used when administration of endotracheal drugs is ineffective
b. is suitable for all crystalloids, colloids and IV drugs
c. should be replaced by IV access as soon as is practical
d. allows aspiration of bone marrow to estimate haemoglobin, but not plasma electrolytes
e. is contraindicated if the limb in which access is being considered is fractured.

Question 7

Adrenaline:

a. is an α_1-agonist
b. is a β_1-agonist
c. is a GABA (gamma-aminobutyric acid) agonist
d. is synthesized by the adrenal cortex
e. is antagonized in patients taking β-blockers.

Question 8

With regard to opioids:

a. all cause respiratory depression
b. fentanyl and alfentanyl are synthetic opioids
c. morphine is broken down into active metabolites
d. naloxone is a partial opioid agonist
e. pethidine is a partial opioid agonist.

Question 9

Ventricular fibrillation:

a. may be triggered by atrial fibrillation
b. may be converted to sinus rhythm by the administration of amiodarone
c. may convert to asystole following defibrillation
d. is associated with worse outcome than asystole when it is the presenting rhythm
e. may be triggered by direct mechanical irritation of the myocardium by an angiogram catheter or guidewire.

Question 10

The adult adrenaline autoinjector (Epipen):

a. delivers 0.5 mg adrenaline in a concentration of 1:1000
b. contains a single dose of adrenaline
c. should be administered into a large forearm vein
d. should be used by a bystander once the patient is unconscious
e. should be stored in the fridge until needed.

Question 11

During external chest compression (ECC) at 100/min, cardiac output is increased by the following:

a. positive end-expiratory pressure (PEEP)
b. increasing the rate of compression.
c. changing rescuers performing ECC every 2 min
d. active decompression
e. ensuring complete chest wall relaxation by removing hands from the chest wall between compressions.

Question 12

Physiological changes during pregnancy include:

a. an increase in blood volume by 20% at term
b. a fall in haematocrit until the end of the second trimester, when levels return towards normal
c. an increase in cardiac output by 40% at term
d. an increase in systemic vascular resistance
e. an increase in respiratory rate and decrease in tidal volume.

Question 13

With regard to VF:

a. the waveform is entirely random
b. a fine waveform is more likely to be cardioverted to a perfusing rhythm than a coarse waveform

c. movement artefact may occasionally be mistaken by an AED for VF
d. the greater the area under the curve with spectral frequency analysis (Fourier analysis), the greater the chances of successful defibrillation
e. the primary determinant of successful defibrillation is the duration of VF.

Question 14

Causes of pulseless electrical activity include:

a. respiratory arrest
b. acute pulmonary embolus, occluding 30% of the pulmonary vascular tree
c. auto-PEEP, as occurs during severe acute asthma
d. calcium channel blocker overdose
e. tricyclic antidepressant overdose.

Question 15

With regard to the ECG:

a. 1 large square $= 0.5$ s
b. the normal PR interval is 0.12 to 0.20 s
c. the normal QRS duration is <0.20 s
d. the normal QT interval (corrected for heart rate; QTc) is $QT/\sqrt{RR}$ (where RR is the interval from the onset of one QRS complex to the onset of the next, measured in seconds)
e. the normal QTc interval is 0.42 s.

Question 16

Automated external defibrillators:

a. have been limited in their use because of difficulties teaching ECG interpretation to lay responders
b. should be used with paediatric pads for children 8 years of age or younger
c. may be used for children <1 year of age if adult pads are not available
d. have sensitivities and specificities for detecting shockable rhythms mostly in excess of 90%
e. have been shown to be ineffective in improving survival from cardiac arrest in the community.

Question 17

Post-resuscitation cooling:

a. risks hypoglycaemia
b. increases the risk of pneumonia
c. causes a mild metabolic alkalosis
d. increases urine output
e. causes hyperkalaemia.

Question 18

Factors favourable for survival from drowning include:

a. water temperature $<5°C$
b. salinated water
c. aspiration of large quantities of water
d. high body mass index
e. young age.

Question 19

Causes of tall T waves on the ECG include:

a. hyperkalaemia
b. hypothermia
c. pulmonary embolus
d. digoxin
e. amiodarone.

Question 20

During external chest compression:

a. myocardial blood flow only occurs during the relaxation phase (diastole)
b. defibrillation is likely to be more successful if delivered during the relaxation phase (diastole)
c. a heart that is still beating is unlikely to be harmed
d. it is recommended that in pregnant women at term, hand position should be slightly higher on the sternum
e. tracheal intubation should not be performed because of risk of trauma to the airway.

Photograph questions

Question 1

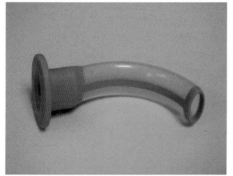

a. What is this?
b. How is it sized?
c. Why is it inserted in adults inverted and then rotated?

Question 2

A patient in a dental chair becomes unresponsive.

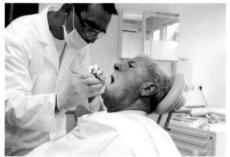

a. What is the most likely cause?
b. What is the treatment?
c. What is the differential diagnosis?

Question 3

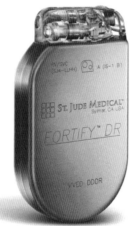

a. What is this implantable device?
b. How may it affect defibrillation electrode position?
c. What are the risks to the rescuer from this device?

Question 4

You are called to the scene to provide medical care for a patient who has been trapped for 3 h by a crush injury to the legs at a serious road traffic accident.

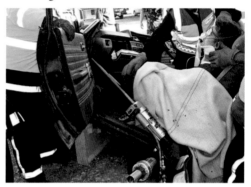

a. What condition may cause collapse of this patient on extrication and why?
b. What treatment on-scene would you consider prior to extrication?
c. What additional hospital therapy may be of benefit?

Question 5

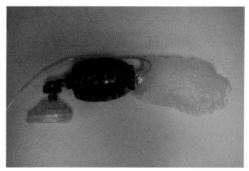

a. What is this device?
b. What is the advantage of a clear face mask?
c. Where should the device be placed during defibrillation?

Diagnostic questions

Question 1

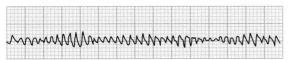

a. What does this rhythm strip show?
b. What conditions are associated with this arrhythmia?
c. What is the treatment of this arrhythmia?

Question 2

a. What rhythm is shown on this ECG rhythm strip?
b. Is a pulse palpable in this patient?
c. What is the treatment?

Question 3

This hypotensive patient has presented to the emergency department with central chest pain radiating to the back.

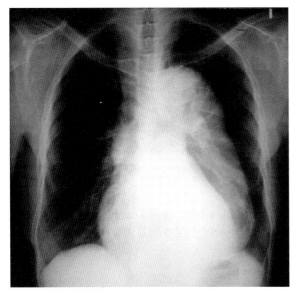

a. What is the likely diagnosis?
b. What imaging investigations are required?
c. What is the treatment?

Question 4

This patient has become short of breath and hypotensive following elective cardiac catheterization. The transthoracic echo is labelled to show the left atrium (LA), left ventricle (LV), right atrium (RA) and right ventricle (RV).

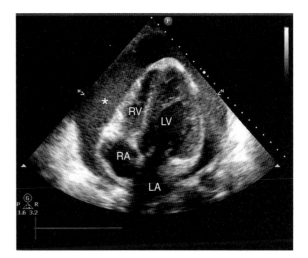

a. What structure is shown as '*'?
b. What is the likely cause of this pathology?
c. What is the treatment?

Question 5

These arterial blood gases are taken from an unconscious patient with an unknown drug overdose:

pH	7.23
Pao_2	13.0 kPa
$Paco_2$	3.8 kPa
HCO_3^-	14.9 mmol/l

a. What is the metabolic condition?
b. What drugs can cause this condition?
c. What other blood tests should be performed?

Short answer questions

Question 1

Draw a biphasic defibrillator waveform, labelling the x and y axes.

Question 2

List the causes of pulseless electrical activity, using the 4Hs and four 4Ts as a guide.

Question 3

List three common drugs causing anaphylaxis.

Question 4

What are the causes of an absent end-tidal CO_2 measurement?

Question 5

A post-arrest patient remains comatose and needs cooling. What methods are available to induce and maintain hypothermia?

MCQ answers

Answer 1

a. **False.** The normal potassium level is 3.5–5.0 mmol/l.
b. **True.**
c. **False.** Hyperkalaemia is exacerbated by acidosis.
d. **True.**
e. **True.**

Answer 2

a. **True.**
b. **False.** Positive pressure ventilation causes increased venous return.
c. **False.** Positive pressure ventilation decreases renal blood flow through decreased cardiac output.
d. **True.** By increasing venous pressure and subsequently the venous drainage of the head.
e. **True.** In patients requiring long-term ventilation.

Answer 3

a. **False.**
b. **True.**
c. **True.** By impairing venous drainage of the head and neck.
d. **False.** Should be fitted in conjunction with airway management.
e. **True.**

Answer 4

a. **True.**
b. **False.**
c. **False.**
d. **False.**
e. **True.** This equation is more accurate than that in (a).

Answer 5

a. **True.**
b. **False.** The palm of the hand represents 1% body surface area.
c. **True.**
d. **True.**
e. **False.** Airway swelling from respiratory tract burns is at its worst 24–48 h after the burn has occurred.

Answer 6

a. **False.** Endotracheal drug route is not recommended. An IO access should be gained promptly if IV cannulation is not possible.
b. **True.**
c. **True.**
d. **False.** Blood and plasma electrolytes can all be measured using bone marrow aspirate.
e. **True.**

Answer 7

a. **True.**
b. **True.**
c. **False.**
d. **False.** Adrenaline is synthesized by chromaffin cells of the adrenal medulla.
e. **True.**

Answer 8

a. **True.**
b. **True.**
c. **True.** Morphine is broken down by glucuronidation to morphine-3,6-diglucuronide, 3-glucuronide and 6-glucuronide; the latter being an opioid agonist.
d. **False.** Naloxone is a pure antagonist.
e. **True.**

Answer 9

a. **False.**
b. **False.** Amiodarone alone will not cardiovert VF. Its membrane-stabilizing effects will increase the efficacy of subsequent defibrillation.
c. **True.**
d. **False.** Patients presenting in asystole have a lower survival rate than those in VF.
e. **True.**

Answer 10

a. **False.** Delivers 0.3 mg adrenaline in a concentration of 1:1000.
b. **True.**
c. **False.** The device is designed to deliver an IM dose; administration of adrenaline IV may cause severe tachyarrhythmias.
d. **False.** Should be used by the patient as soon as he or she become symptomatic.
e. **False.** Should be kept with the patient at all times.

19

Answer 11

a. **False.** PEEP will increase intrathoracic impedance and reduce venous return, which reduces subsequent cardiac output.
b. **False.** A rate of 100–120/min is considered optimal to allow adequate myocardial filling between compressions.
c. **True.** Rescuer fatigue occurs after just 2 min of ECC.
d. **True.** Active decompression (e.g. suction cup applied to the chest wall to actively lift the chest wall during the relaxation phase of chest compression) will increase cardiac output, although this has not been shown in clinical studies to improve survival.
e. **True.**

Answer 12

a. **False.** Blood volume increases by 45–50% at term.
b. **True.**
c. **True.**
d. **False.** Systemic vascular resistance falls markedly as pregnancy progresses.
e. **False.** Respiratory rate increases slightly and tidal volume increases 40% at term.

Answer 13

a. **False.** The VF waveform is not entirely random, having a degree of predictability.
b. **False.** A coarse rhythm is more likely to be cardioverted successfully.
c. **True.** There are a number of case reports of automatic defibrillators mistaking movement artefact (vibration in an ambulance) for a shockable rhythm.
d. **True.**
e. **True.**

Answer 14

a. **True.** The commonest cause of pulseless electrical activity, being implicated as the cause in 25–53% of cases.
b. **False.** Over 50% of the pulmonary vascular tree needs to be occluded to cause haemodynamic collapse.

c. **True.** Auto-PEEP occurs in acute asthma when air trapping results in hyperinflation of the lungs. Auto-PEEP may exceed 80 cmH$_2$O in severe cases, with the resulting increase in intrathoracic pressure impairing venous return and the hyperinflated lungs compressing the heart, to prevent filling.
d. **True.** Calcium channel blockers can depress myocardial function and cause haemodynamic collapse.
e. **True.** Tricyclic antidepressants can depress myocardial function and cause haemodynamic collapse.

Answer 15

a. **False.** 1 large square = 0.2 s.
b. **True.**
c. **False.** The normal QRS duration is <0.12 s.
d. **True.**
e. **True.**

Answer 16

a. **False.** Although some AEDs may have an ECG display, interpretation of this display is unnecessary because the AED software will analyse the arrhythmia and advise a shock if appropriate.
b. **True.**
c. **True.**
d. **True.**
e. **False.** Several studies have shown that AEDs can increase survival in the community when sufficient numbers of trained responders and short geographic distances allow quick response times.

Answer 17

a. **False.** Hypothermia decreases insulin sensitivity and reduces insulin secretion by pancreatic islet cells, risking hyperglycaemia.
b. **True.**
c. **False.** Causes a mild metabolic acidosis.
d. **True.**
e. **False.** Causes hypokalaemia.
(See Deakin CD *et al. Resuscitation*, 2010;81:1305–1352.)

Answer 18

a. **True.**
b. **False.** Salinity of water does not affect survival.
c. **True.** Aspiration of large quantities of water helps to induce rapid cooling.
d. **False.** Obese patients (high body mass index) have excess adipose tissue, which acts as an insulator and limits rapid cooling.
e. **True.**

Answer 19

a. **True.**
b. **False.**
c. **False.**
d. **False.** Digoxin tends to cause flattened T waves.
e. **False.**

Answer 20

a. **False.** Unlike the beating heart, myocardial blood flow occurs during both systole and diastole.
b. **True.**
c. **True.** Although some studies have suggested a greater risk of inducing VF.
d. **True.**
e. **False.** When possible, tracheal intubation should be performed without interruption to external chest compression.

Photograph answers

Answer 1

a. This is an oropharyngeal (Guedel) airway.
b. It is sized by measuring against the patient's head: the flange is aligned with the incisors and the tip to the tragus of the ear.

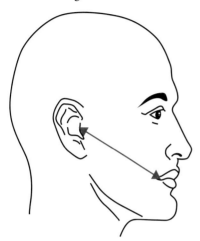

c. The Guedel airway is inserted inverted in order to avoid catching the tongue and pushing it backwards during insertion. Once contact is made with the back of the throat, the airway is rotated 180°, allowing for easy insertion.

Answer 2

a. A vasovagal collapse (faint) is the commonest cause of collapse in the dental chair. Also consider anaphylaxis, myocardial infarction.
b. Stop any stimulation, elevate the legs and give O_2.
c. Other less common causes of collapse include anaphylaxis, arrhythmia or cardiac arrest.

Answer 3

a. Automatic implantable cardioverter–defibrillator (AICD).
b. Defibrillation pads or paddles should be placed at least 8 cm away from this device to avoid escape current damaging the device or being transmitted down the defibrillation electrode to damage the myocardium.

c. The discharge from an AICD may cause pectoral muscle contraction in the patient, and shocks to the rescuer have been documented. In view of the low energy levels discharged by AICDs (<40 J), it is unlikely that any significant harm will be caused to the rescuer, but the wearing of gloves and minimizing contact with the patient while the device is discharging is prudent.

Answer 4

a. Patients with limbs trapped for >30 min are at risk of crush syndrome. This results from ischaemic damage to limbs, with subsequent reperfusion injury, and appears after the release of the crushing pressure. The mechanism is believed to be rhabdomyolysis (muscle breakdown caused by ischaemia) leading to the release into the bloodstream of breakdown products (e.g. myoglobin, potassium and phosphorus).
b. Prior to extrication, consider a saline infusion of 1000–1500 ml/h, initiated during extrication. Sodium bicarbonate should also be considered in these patients at the time of extrication. Consider gradual release of the entrapped limb to limit the sudden release of toxins.
c. Forced alkaline diuresis, up to 8 l/24 h, should be maintained (urine pH >6.5). Alkalinization increases the urine solubility of haematin and aids in its excretion. This should be continued until myoglobin is no longer detectable in the urine. Mannitol may also be of benefit, both as a scavenger of oxygen free radicals and through its actions as an osmotic diuretic.

Answer 5

a. Self-inflating bag-valve-mask.
b. Allows the rescuer to see any blood or vomit coming from the mouth or nose.
c. At least 1 m away from the patient.

Diagnostic answers

Answer 1

a. Torsade de pointes. Torsade is a polymorphic ventricular tachycardia in which the morphology of the QRS complexes varies from beat to beat. The ventricular rate ranges from 150 to 250/min. Because it is associated with regular variation of the morphology of the QRS vector from positive to net negative and back again, it was termed torsade de pointes, or 'twisting of the point', about the isoelectric axis.

b. Brugada syndrome, Jervell syndrome, Lange–Nielsen syndrome and the Romano–Ward syndrome. Also Takotsubo cardiomyopathy (stress-induced cardiomyopathy).

c. Stop amiodarone, which may worsen the condition. Administer magnesium sulphate 2–4 g IV. Magnesium is usually very effective, even in a patient with a normal magnesium level. Other therapies include overdrive pacing and isoprenaline infusion. Patients in extremis should be treated with electrical cardioversion.

Answer 2

a. Acute aortic dissection.

b. Transoesophageal echocardiogram, CT angiogram (or MRI) of the heart and aorta.

c. Surgical repair or occasionally endovascular stenting may be possible.

Answer 3

a. P wave asystole.

b. There is no cardiac output and, therefore, no pulse.

c. Cardiac arrest ALS algorithm for non-shockable arrhythmias.

Answer 4

a. Fluid in the pericardial space (i.e. cardiac tamponade).

b. Perforation of the right atrium or right ventricle by the catheter.

c. Insertion of a pericardial drain to relieve the tamponade and possible surgery if the bleeding continues.

Answer 5

a. Uncompensated (acute) metabolic acidosis.

b. Salicylate (aspirin) intoxication, methanol, ethylene glycol, toluene (a solvent).

c. Blood levels should also be checked for paracetamol levels. Paracetamol is commonly taken as an overdose, either separately or combined with salicylate.

Short answers

Answer 1

There are two main biphasic waveforms, both shown below:

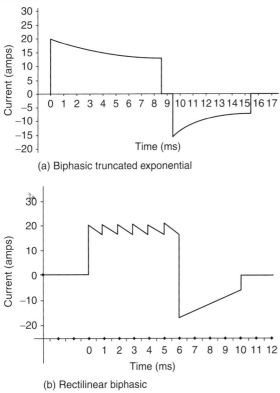

(a) Biphasic truncated exponential

(b) Rectilinear biphasic

Answer 2

4Hs:

- hypovolaemia
- hypoxia
- hypokalaemia/hyperkalaemia
- hypothermia.

4Ts:

- toxins
- tamponade (cardiac)
- thrombosis (pulmonary or coronary)
- tension pneumothorax.

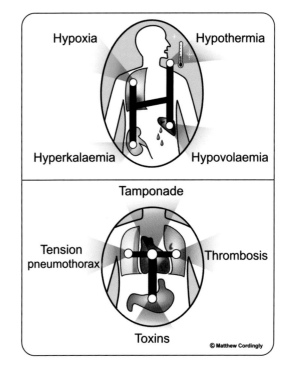

Answer 3

Drug types causing anaphylaxis:

- antibiotics: penicillin, cephalosporins (particularly first generation such as cefalotin, cefalexin, cefadroxil and cefazolin)
- neuromuscular blockers (e.g. vecuronium, pancuronium)
- anaesthetic induction agents (e.g. thiopental, propofol)
- opioids (morphine)
- non-steroidal anti-inflammatory drugs
- colloids
- IV radiocontrast media.

Answer 4

Causes:

- faulty/disconnected capnography or breathing circuit
- oesophageal intubation
- loss of cardiac output
- cessation of ventilation.

Answer 5

Initial cooling is facilitated by neuromuscular blockade and sedation, which will prevent shivering. Magnesium sulphate reduces the shivering threshold.

External methods:

- simple ice packs and/or wet towels
- cooling blankets or pads
- water or air circulating blankets
- water circulating gel-coated pads.

Internal methods:

- infusion of 30 ml/kg of 4°C saline or Hartmann's solution decreases core temperature by approximately 1.5°C (induction of hypothermia only)
- intravascular heat exchanger, usually placed in the femoral or subclavian vein
- cardiopulmonary bypass.

Multiple choice questions

Question 1

With regard to hyperkalaemia:

a. acute hyperkalaemia is less well tolerated than chronic hyperkalaemia
b. glucose and insulin given together result in potassium uptake into cells
c. calcium IV may protect against harmful effects
d. all diuretics increase potassium loss and may lower potassium levels
e. renal dialysis may be indicated if severe.

Question 2

With regard to endotracheal tube size:

a. adult sizes are usually appropriate for patients aged >16 years
b. the appropriate size of a paediatric uncuffed tube is given by the equation $(Age/4) + 4$
c. the appropriate size of a paediatric cuffed tube is given by the equation $(Age/4) + 3$
d. tracheostomy tubes should be 1.0 mm smaller than the corresponding endotracheal tube size
e. tubes of smaller internal diameter reduce airway resistance.

Question 3

With regard to paediatric fluid resuscitation:

a. a paediatric fluid bolus is generally calculated as 20–30 ml/kg
b. maintenance fluids can be calculated using the 4-2-1 rule,
   • 0–10 kg: 4 ml/kg per h
   • 10–20 kg: +2 ml/kg per h
   • >20 kg: 1 ml/kg per h
c. Children have higher body water content than adults

d. children with 15–20% dehydration have physical findings that include tenting of the skin, weight loss, sunken eyes and fontanel, slight lethargy and dry mucous membranes
e. crystalloids rather than colloids are the fluid of choice for volume resuscitation.

Question 4

Causes of a short PR interval include:

a. Wolff–Parkinson–White syndrome
b. Lown–Ganong–Levine syndrome
c. Duchenne muscular dystrophy
d. Type II glycogen storage disease (Pompe disease)
e. ischaemic cardiomyopathy.

Question 5

With regard to electrical safety during external defibrillation:

a. paddles are safer than self-adhesive pads
b. clinical gloves may reduce the risk of an inadvertent shock to the rescuer
c. sources of O_2 should be turned off during defibrillation
d. electrode paste reduces the risk of arcing between electrodes
e. 24% O_2 doubles the rate of combustion.

Question 6

Whole bowel irrigation for drug overdose:

a. is particularly effective for late presenting paracetamol or aspirin overdose
b. is an alternative to combined laxative and emetic therapy
c. may be considered for toxic ingestions of sustained-release or enteric-coated drugs
d. is contraindicated in patients with hypothermia
e. is contraindicated in patients with haemodynamic instability.

Question 7

In the management of anaphylaxis:

a. the α-agonist actions of adrenaline reverse peripheral vasodilation
b. the β-agonist actions of adrenaline suppress histamine release
c. the adult dose of adrenaline is 0.5 mg IM
d. the adrenaline dose for children 6–12 years is 0.3 mg IM
e. adrenaline IM should be administered at 15 min intervals until an improvement is seen.

Question 8

With regard to resuscitation during pregnancy:

a. the gravid uterus obstructs inferior vena caval blood flow from approximately 40 weeks of gestation
b. manual displacement of the uterus to the left should be performed before attempting lateral tilt
c. a tracheal tube 0.5–1.0 mm smaller than usual may be required because of laryngeal oedema
d. increased transthoracic impedance means that external defibrillation should be performed using the highest defibrillator energy settings possible
e. external chest compressions should be performed over the upper one-third of the sternum.

Question 9

Paediatric cardiac arrest:

a. is most commonly from hypoxia-related causes rather than primary cardiac pathology
b. presents with asystole in approximately 80% of out-of-hospital cases
c. in hospital, most commonly is caused by respiratory pathology
d. has sudden infant death syndrome (SIDS) as its leading cause
e. can be accurately diagnosed by healthcare professionals using a pulse check.

Question 10

Causes of flattened T waves on the ECG include:

a. pulmonary embolus
b. right bundle branch block
c. left bundle branch block
d. pericarditis
e. digoxin effect.

Question 11

Risks to rescuers during CPR are:

a. induction of VF caused by accidental contact with the patient during defibrillation
b. HIV infection from needlestick injury
c. infection with swine flu through droplet spread
d. reduced by using a barrier device for mouth-to-mouth ventilation
e. a cause of poor rates of bystander CPR.

Question 12

When summoning help at a cardiac arrest:

a. a 'crash call' number is the internal hospital telephone number dialled to summon the emergency team following a cardiac arrest in hospital
b. 222 is the standard number for assistance in UK hospitals
c. 911 is the officially designated emergency telephone number in Canada and the USA
d. 112 is the European emergency number in use across the European Union
e. police and fire are usually accessed using different numbers to 911 or 112.

Question 13

Causes of low-amplitude ECG complexes include:

a. poor lead connection
b. lead electrodes placed too close together
c. obesity
d. left or right ventricular hypertrophy
e. myocardial stunning following defibrillation.

Question 14

Central venous catheters (CVCs):

a. when coated with chlorhexidine may be a cause of anaphylaxis.
b. are less of an infection risk when placed in the internal jugular vein than when placed in the femoral vein
c. require antibiotic prophylaxis to cover insertion
d. are at greatest risk of causing a pneumothorax when placed in the internal jugular vein
e. inserted by subcutaneous tunnelling reduces the incidence of catheter infection.

Question 15

Cardiac arrest in electrocution:

a. is usually associated with higher voltages in adults than children
b. may occur as a result of respiratory arrest
c. may be caused by coronary artery spasm induced by the electric current
d. is more likely with hand–foot current pathways than hand–hand pathways
e. is a greater risk with moist skin, which decreases electrical resistance.

Question 16

Naloxone:

a. can be administered by IV, IM, subcutaneous (SC), IO or intranasal (IN) routes
b. has an initial adult dose of 400 μg by any route
c. has a duration of action of approximately 60 min
d. in large opioid overdoses may require titration of naloxone to a total dose of 6–10 mg
e. administration in chronic opioid abusers may cause acute withdrawal symptoms and is contraindicated.

Question 17

Causes of cardiac arrest in asthma include:

a. hyperventilation causing respiratory alkalosis
b. severe bronchospasm and mucous plugging leading to asphyxia
c. tension pneumothorax
d. arrhythmias triggered by hypoxia
e. raised intrathoracic pressure (caused by auto-PEEP: gas trapped in the airways exerting a positive pressure) impairing venous return and subsequent cardiac output.

Question 18

Hypermagnesaemia may present as:

a. confusion
b. weakness
c. respiratory failure
d. cardiac arrest
e. hyperglycaemia.

Question 19

Urine alkalinization:

a. requires a blood pH of 7.5 or higher
b. is a first line treatment for moderate-to-severe salicylate poisoning in patients who do not need haemodialysis
c. may cause hyperkalaemia
d. may be effective in some forms of herbicide poisoning
e. is induced using an IV bicarbonate infusion.

Question 20

With regard to the management of electrical injury:

a. compartment syndrome, cardiac arrhythmias or myoglobinuria is uncommon in patients exposed to less than 500 V (low voltage)
b. patients found in VF may have no external signs of burn
c. high-voltage alternating current (AC) often causes rapid muscle contraction that throws the victim away from the source, minimizing duration of electrical contact
d. taser barbs from police weapons discharging into the chest wall may induce VF
e. sudden death from VF is more common with low-voltage AC, whereas asystole is more often associated with high-voltage AC or DC.

Photograph questions

Question 1

a. What does this sign indicate?
b. Where is it likely to be found?
c. What training is required for a member of the public to use an AED?

Question 2

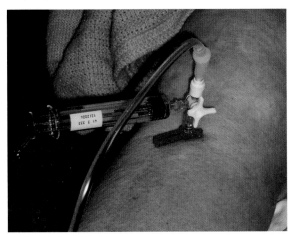

a. What device has been inserted into this patient's tibia?
b. What causes pain on injection of fluids or drugs through this device.
c. What is the effect of lignocaine given through this device on the pain of subsequent infusions?

Question 3

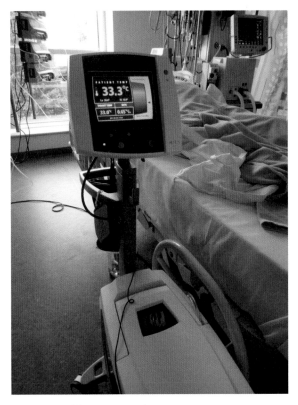

a. What is this device?
b. What are the indications for cooling post-arrest?
c. What is the target core temperature and duration for a period of therapeutic hypothermia?

Question 4

A patient receiving a blood transfusion becomes wheezy and hypotensive during the first 30 min of a blood transfusion.

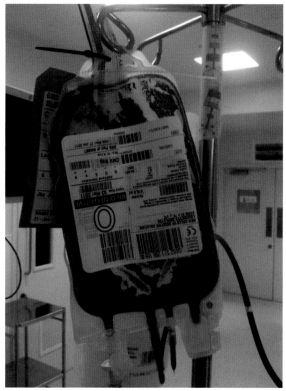

a. What are the two most likely causes?
b. What is the immediate treatment?
c. Why is this unlikely to be transfusion-related acute lung injury (TRALI)?

Question 5

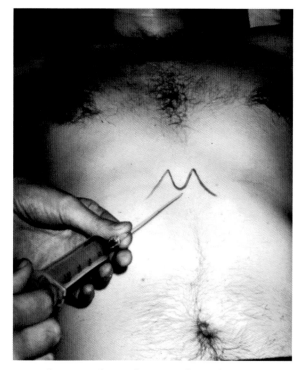

a. What procedure is being performed?
b. What are the landmarks and needle direction for this procedure?
c. What indicates accidental intraventricular rather than pericardial needle placement?

Diagnostic questions

Question 1

The following arterial blood gas sample, from a normal patient breathing room air, has been drawn from an arterial line. What is the likely diagnosis?

Hb	10.1 g/dl (101 g/l)
pH	7.39
Pa_{O_2}	15.7 kPa
Pa_{CO_2}	3.5 kPa
HCO_3^-	22.3 mmol/l

Question 2

A member of the resuscitation team receives a needle-stick injury from a patient during a resuscitation attempt. The patient's blood shows the following serology:

- hepatitis B 'e' antigen titre: **low**
- hepatitis B 's' antigen titre: **high**.

a. Is the rescuer at risk of being infected by hepatitis B virus and why?
b. What treatment is required?

Question 5

a. What rhythm does this ECG show?
b. What is the treatment?

Question 3

A 64-year-old patient presents with chest pain in the emergency department. The ECG is shown below in question 5. What are the immediate priorities in treating this patient?

Question 4

A routine blood sample shows the following results:

Na^+	131 mmol/l
K^+	2.9 mmol/l
urea	5.4 mmol/l
creatinine	120 mmol/l

The patient is taking the following drugs:

atenolol	50 mg PO once daily (o.d.)
ramipril	5 mg PO o.d.
furosemide	80 mg PO o.d.
aspirin	75 mg PO o.d.

What is the most likely cause of the hypokalaemia and why?

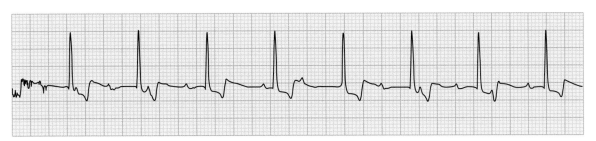

Short answer questions

Question 1

What is the treatment for inadvertent intra-arterial injection of a vasoconstrictor?

Question 2

Draw a monophasic defibrillation waveform and label the x and y axes.

Question 3

Discuss the immediate management of Paraquat poisoning

Question 4

What are the causes of a metabolic acidosis that may lead to a cardiac arrest?

Question 5

Why does the paediatric BLS algorithm commence with ventilations, but the adult BLS algorithm commence with chest compressions?

MCQ answers

Answer 1

a. **True**.

b. **True**.

c. **True**. However, there is no scientific evidence for the benefit of calcium in hyperkalaemia.

d. **False**. Although most diuretics increase K^+ excretion, some such as spironolactone are potassium sparing and may cause hyperkalaemia.

e. **True**.

Answer 2

a. **True**.

b. **True**.

c. **True**.

d. **False**.

e. **False**. Larger internal diameter tubes reduce airway resistance.

Answer 3

a. **True**.

b. **True**.

c. **True**. Water makes up approximately 70% of body weight in infants, 65% in children and 60% in adults.

d. **False**. The physical findings are present with no more than 6–10% fluid loss.

e. **False**. In a 2004 *Cochrane Database Review*, investigators examined a series of randomized trials of colloids compared with crystalloids in patients who required volume replacement. There was no evidence to favour one type of fluid over the other (Roberts I *et al. Cochrane Database Syst Rev*, 2004;(4):CD000567).

Answer 4

a. **True**.

b. **True**.

c. **True**.

d. **True**.

e. **False**. Tends to cause a prolonged PR interval.

Answer 5

a. **False**. Self-adhesive pads provide better contact with the skin and may reduce the risk of arcing between electrodes.

b. **True**. Although latex and non-latex gloves tend to disintegrate at relatively low currents and are often torn during resuscitation.

c. **False**. Sources of O_2 should be at least 1 m away from the patient.

d. **False**. Electrode paste may smear over the chest wall and increase the risk of arcing between electrodes. Its use is no longer recommended.

e. **True**.

Answer 6

a. **False**.

b. **False**. Laxatives and/or emetics have no role in the acute management of drug overdose.

c. **Talse**.

d. **False**.

e. **True**.

Answer 7

a. **True**.

b. **True**.

c. **True**.

d. **True**.

e. **False**. Adrenaline is recommended to be given every 5 min until improvement is seen.

Answer 8

a. **False**. Obstruction is thought to occur from approximately 20 weeks of gestation.

b. **True**. Manual uterine displacement can be performed quickly and easily. Lateral tilt is more difficult to perform, usually requires a wedge and may make external chest compression less effective.

c. **True**.

d. **False**. There is no significant change in transthoracic impedance during pregnancy and standard defibrillation energy settings should be used.

e. **False**. Although previous guidelines have suggested that a higher than usual hand position is required, there is no evidence to support this recommendation and standard hand positioning is recommended.

Answer 9

a. **True.** Paediatric cardiac arrest is uncommon; progressive respiratory failure accounts for 60% of all paediatric arrests.

b. **True.** Asystole has been documented in 78.9% cases, followed by pulseless electrical activity (13.5%) and VF (3.8%) (Kuisma M *et al. Resuscitation*, 1995;30:141–150).

c. **False.** Cardiovascular causes of cardiac arrest are the most common (41% of all arrests), with hypovolaemia from blood loss and hyperkalaemia from transfusion of stored blood the most common cardiovascular causes. Among respiratory causes of arrest (27%), airway obstruction from laryngospasm is the most common. Medication-related arrests account for 18% of all arrests. Vascular injury incurred during placement of central venous catheters is the most common equipment-related cause of arrest (Bhananker SM, *et al. Anesth Analg*, 2007;105:344–350).

d. **False.** SIDS is the leading cause of paediatric cardiac arrest, followed by trauma, airway-related cardiac arrest and (near) drowning.

e. **False.** In the paediatric studies, healthcare professionals are able to accurately detect a pulse by palpation only 80% of the time and mistakenly perceive a pulse when it is actually absent in approximately 20% of cases.

Answer 10

a. **True.**
b. **True.**
c. **False.**
d. **True.**
e. **True.**

Answer 11

a. **False.** This has never been documented in the literature.
b. **True.**
c. **True.**
d. **True.**
e. **True.**

Answer 12

a. **True.**
b. **False.** The standard hospital number is 2222.
c. **True.**
d. **True.**
e. **False.** 911 or 112 are used to access all emergency services.

Answer 13

a. **False.**
b. **True.**
c. **True.**
d. **False.**
e. **False.**

Answer 14

a. **True.**
b. **True.**
c. **False.**
d. **False.** The subclavian route is the highest risk for a pneumothorax as the tip of the needle may puncture the pleura over the apex of the lung.
e. **True.** Subcutaneous tunnelling of short-term CVCs is thought to reduce the incidence of catheter infection by increasing the distance between the venous entry site and skin emergence.

Answer 15

a. **True.** Adult electrocution tends to occur more commonly at work, in association with higher industrial voltages, whereas children tend to be electrocuted with domestic voltages (110–240 V).

b. **True.** Respiratory arrest may be caused by paralysis of the respiratory centre or the respiratory muscles themselves.

c. **True.** Coronary artery spasm may result in myocardial ischaemia and subsequent cardiac arrest.

d. **False.** Hand–hand pathways result in more current traversing the myocardium compared with hand–foot pathways, and are more likely to induce cardiac arrest.

e. **True.**

Answer 16

a. **True.**

b. **False.** The initial doses of naloxone are 400 μg IV/IO, 800 μg IM, 800 μg SC or 2 mg IN.

c. **True.** Respiratory depression can persist for 4–5 h after opioid overdose, so repeated naloxone doses may be necessary.

d. **True.**

e. **False.** Although naloxone may cause acute withdrawal, its administration is not contraindicated in chronic opioid abusers.

Answer 17

a. **False.** Asthma causes hypoventilation with progressive respiratory and metabolic acidosis.

b. **True.**

c. **True.**

d. **True.**

e. **True.**

Answer 18

a. **True.**

b. **True.**

c. **True.**

d. **True.**

e. **True.**

Answer 19

a. **False.** Requires a urine pH of 7.5 or higher.

b. **True.**

c. **False.** Hypokalaemia is the commonest electrolyte disturbance.

d. **True.** For the herbicides 2,4-dichlorophenoxyacetic acid and methylchlorophenoxypropionic acid (Mecoprop).

e. **True.**

Answer 20

a. **True.** Although, patients sustaining burns from 200–1000 V may have significant local tissue destruction.

b. **True.** As relatively little current is required to induce arrythmias. VF can occur at currents of 50–100 mA.

c. **False.** High-voltage DC often causes rapid muscle contraction, which throws the victim away from the source and minimizes duration of electrical contact. In contrast, AC of the same voltage is considered to be more dangerous because it causes tetanic muscle contractions, which render the victim unable to release their hand from the electrical contact.

d. **False.** Tasers deliver high-voltage current through a series of DC shocks. They deliver 50 000 V, with an average current of 2.1 mA. Studies in healthy volunteers have failed to demonstrate arrhythmias or cardiac damage.

e. **True.**

Photograph answers

Answer 1

a. This is the International Liaison Committee on Resuscitation universal sign to indicate the presence of an AED, the localization of an AED in a room, a container with an AED for public use or the direction to follow in order to reach the AED. Its purpose is to assist in the rapid identification of an AED in cases of cardiac arrest.

b. Public places with large public gatherings such as shopping centres, airports, railway stations, ferries, passenger planes and gyms.

c. In the UK, there are no legal requirements for users to have had any training in order to use an AED.

Answer 2

a. Intraosseous needle.

b. Pain on injection results from an increased pressure within the bone marrow. It is, therefore, related to the rate at which fluids are injected; the slower the rate, the less the pain.

c. Although lignocaine has been advocated as an effective way of reducing pain on injection through an intraosseous needle, it is ineffective as it has no effect on stretch receptors in the bone marrow.

Answer 3

a. Alsius CoolGard/Zoll Thermoguard Management device. (An intravascular countercurrent cooling device controlled through this trolley.)

b. Unconscious adult patients with spontaneous circulation after out-of-hospital VF cardiac arrest. Cooling should be considered for other rhythms or in-hospital cardiac arrest.

c. Patients should be cooled to 32–34°C for 12 to 24 h when the initial rhythm was VF. Such cooling may also be beneficial for other rhythms or in-hospital cardiac arrest.

Answer 4

a. Acute haemolytic transfusion reaction or severe allergic reaction/anaphylaxis.

b. Stop the transfusion, then:
   - check the patient's identity and recheck against details on blood unit and compatibility label
   - give O_2 and IV fluids as appropriate
   - consider hydrocortisone 200 mg IV and chlorphenamine 10–20 mg IV
   - if hypotension is severe, give adrenaline 0.5–1 mg IM and repeat every 10 min until improvement occurs.

c. TRALI is characterized by acute respiratory distress and bilaterally symmetrical pulmonary oedema with hypoxaemia developing within 2 to 8 h after a transfusion.

Answer 5

a. Needle pericardiocentesis.

b. The needle is inserted below the xiphisternum and directed towards the tip of the left scapula. The needle track is at a 45° angle to the abdominal wall and 45° away from the midline, as shown. Where possible, needle insertion should be performed under direct ultrasound guidance.

c. Indications:
   - intracardiac blood forms a clot, whereas pericardial aspirate does not usually form a clot
   - the pericardial aspirate should usually have a lower haemoglobin level than the patient's peripheral blood
   - widening of the QRS complex, ST segment changes or multiple ventricular dysrrhythmias, indicate myocardial puncture
   - unlimited aspiration of blood without clinical improvement indicates ventricular aspiration.

Diagnostic answers

Answer 1

This sample has low haemoglobin, normal pH, an elevated Pao_2 and a lowered $Paco_2$. These changes are typical of accidental dilution with heparin. The pH will not change because of the large buffering capacity of haemoglobin and plasma proteins. The Pao_2 will rise, while $Paco_2$ decreases: changes occurring in proportion to the relative differences in partial pressure of these gases between blood and the heparin. The lowered haemoglobin is a result of haemodilution.

Answer 2

Hepatitis B 'e' antigen is a viral protein present in hepatitis B-infected cells. It is present in patients with acute or chronic hepatitis B infections. It is a marker of active viral disease and the degree of infectiousness of the patient. Titres lag behind those of hepatitis B 's' antigen (surface antigen). Hepatitis B 's' antigen appears early in the disease, peaks with the onset of symptoms and disappears 6 months post-infection. Patients who are positive for hepatitis B 's' antigen are considered infectious.

a. The serology suggests that the patient has an active hepatitis B infection and is, therefore, at risk of infecting recipients.
b. If the individual with the needlestick injury has high levels of hepatitis B surface antibody (usually resulting from hepatitis B vaccination), they are considered immune to the hepatitis B virus. An individual with low hepatitis B surface antibody levels may require immediate hepatitis B vaccination, and hepatitis B immunoglobulin should be considered. Screening should also be undertaken for HIV.

Answer 3

High-flow O_2, aspirin 300 mg PO (unless contraindicated), glyceryl trinitrate (GTN) 400 µg sublingually, analgesia (morphine boluses, 1–2 mg IV, titrated against pain), alerting the duty cardiologist to review the patient with possible need for percutaneous coronary intervention (PCI). Consider 300 mg clopidogrel PO and unfractionated heparin (or a derivative, e.g. Fondaparinux), according to local protocol.

Answer 4

Furosemide (a loop diuretic) prevents the reabsorption of Na^+ and Cl^- chloride ions at the loop of Henle in the kidney. As a result, more Na^+ and chloride reach the distal tubule and collecting duct. Here, Na^+ is reabsorbed in exchange for K^+; the increased Na^+ load resulting in increased K^+ excretion. Hydrogen ions are also exchanged for Na^+, resulting in a metabolic alkalosis.

Answer 5

a. Complete heart block (third-degree heart block).
b. A trial of atropine may be considered, but it is usually ineffective and a temporary or permanent pacemaker is the treatment of choice.

Short answers

Answer 1

- Stop drug administration and if possible aspirate from the cannula to reduce the amount of drug present in the tissues (leave the cannula in place for saline irrigation if indicated).
- Elevate the limb to reduce swelling and promote venous drainage.
- Heat may promote vasodilatation and increase drug reabsorption and distribution.
- Also consider the following:
  - saline washout
  - liposuction
  - steroids
  - hyaluronidase
  - phentolamine
  - regional sympathetic block.
  - (For a good review, see Lake C, Beecroft CL *Contin Educ Anaesth Crit Care Pain*, 2010;10:109–113.)

Answer 2

Monophasic damped sinusoidal (MDS) waveform:

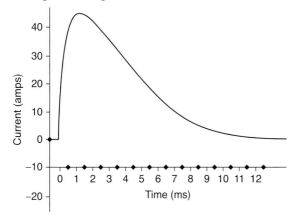

Answer 3

There is no specific treatment for Paraquat poisoning. The aims are to relieve symptoms and treat complications as they arise:

- remove all contaminated clothing
- gently wash any contaminated skin with soap and water for 15 min (hard scrubbing risks abrasions, which may increase absorption)
- give activated charcoal if oral absorption has occurred
- consider haemoperfusion for sicker patients
- do not routinely give supplementary O_2, which worsens pulmonary fibrosis; only give O_2 to maintain adequate O_2 saturations if necessary.

Answer 4

Causes of metabolic acidosis include:

- lactic acidosis
- ketoacidosis
- intoxication:
  - salicylates
  - ethanol
  - methanol
  - formaldehyde
  - ethylene glycol
  - paraldehyde
- massive rhabdomyolysis
- intoxication:
  - ammonium chloride
  - acetazolamide (Diamox)
  - toluene
  - isopropyl alcohol
  - glue sniffing.

Answer 5

Unlike adults, paediatric cardiac arrest is usually caused by hypoxaemia. Giving rescue breaths before chest compressions ensures that oxygenated blood is circulated when the chest compressions commence. Commencing with chest compressions would only circulate deoxygenated blood.

Multiple choice questions

Question 1

ECG changes of hyperkalaemia include:

a. increased PR interval
b. prominent U waves
c. inverted T waves
d. reduced R wave amplitude
e. increased QRS duration.

Question 2

Causes of a prolonged PR interval include:

a. first-degree heart block
b. second-degree heart block (Mobitz type I)
c. second-degree heart block (Mobitz type II)
d. third-degree heart block
e. atrial fibrillation.

Question 3

When rewarming a patient suffering from severe accidental hypothermia:

a. if the core temperature is less than 30°C, IV resuscitation drugs should be given every 6–10 min rather than the standard 3–5 min
b. warm IV fluids (40°C) are an effective method of initiating rewarming
c. active internal rewarming techniques include gastric, peritoneal, pleural or bladder lavage with warmed fluids at 60°C
d. in a hypothermic patient with cardiac arrest, extracorporeal rewarming is the preferred method of active internal rewarming
e. during rewarming, patients will require large volumes of IV fluids as vasodilation causes expansion of the intravascular space.

Question 4

The atrioventricular node of the heart:

a. stimulates the sinoatrial node during normal sinus rhythm
b. discharges through the bundle of His.
c. conducts more slowly the faster it is stimulated
d. has an intrinsic firing rate of 40–60/min
e. is stimulated directly by the ventricular lead of a pacemaker.

Question 5

The impedance threshold valve (ITD):

a. generates a negative intrathoracic pressure during passive chest recoil
b. decreases venous return
c. increases spontaneous cardiac output
d. is not recommended to be used with supraglottic airway devices
e. is indicated for cardiac arrest of all aetiology.

Question 6

External chest compressions:

a. should be performed at a rate of 100–120/min in adults
b. should be performed at a rate of 100–120/min in children
c. may be more effective when performed on a hospital mattress
d. may induce arrhythmias when performed on a patient in sinus rhythm
e. may be more effective when rate is maintained using a metronome.

Question 7

Myocardial blood flow during CPR:

a. is determined by coronary perfusion pressure: the difference in aortic and right atrial pressure
b. occurs during both the compression and decompression phases of external chest compression
c. may be reversed if venous pressures are high
d. remains constant during good-quality CPR
e. is low because coronary perfusion pressures are only 10–20 mmHg (compared with a threshold of 40–60 mmHg to generate adequate flow).

Question 8

Atrial fibrillation (AF):

a. is defined as 'paroxysmal' if recurrent episodes self-terminate in fewer than 7 days
b. doubles the risk of stroke if untreated
c. may occur secondary to carbon monoxide poisoning
d. may respond to unsynchronized electrical cardioversion
e. usually results from electrical foci arising from myocytes in and around the base of the pulmonary veins.

Question 9

Torsade de pointes:

a. is a polymorphic ventricular tachycardia
b. may progress to VF
c. may be treated with synchronized cardioversion
d. is more common in malnourished individuals and chronic alcoholics
e. may be precipitated by some antiarrhythmic drugs such as sotalol, procainamide and quinidine.

Question 10

Monophasic waveforms:

a. are extended in duration in patients with high transthoracic impedance
b. should be delivered at 360 J for all ventricular arrhythmias
c. have been shown to be less effective than biphasic waveforms in achieving survival to hospital discharge
d. may deliver up to 5000 V
e. cause more severe cutaneous burns than biphasic waveforms.

Question 11

Bystander CPR:

a. increases survival to hospital discharge rates by 50%
b. is undertaken in 60–70% of out-of-hospital cardiac arrests
c. is more commonly performed when the rescuer does not know the victim

d. should be undertaken without the mouth-to-mouth component if the bystander is unwilling to perform this
e. should not be performed in traumatic cardiac arrest.

Question 12

With regards to opioid overdose:

a. heroin is an opioid
b. diamorphine is the same drug as heroin
c. diamorphine is metabolized to morphine
d. morphine is more lipid soluble than diamorphine so it is absorbed more rapidly across mucous membranes
e. methadone is a partial opioid agonist.

Question 13

The Lund University Cardiac Assist System (LUCAS) device:

a. is battery powered
b. uses active decompression
c. compresses at a rate of 100/min
d. allows defibrillation during chest compression
e. can be used during percutaneous coronary intervention.

Question 14

Hypocalcaemia may be caused by:

a. metabolic acidosis
b. calcium channel blocker overdose
c. hypothermia
d. asphyxial cardiac arrest
e. rhabdomyolysis.

Question 15

Adrenaline:

a. is given after the third cycle of CPR for non-shockable rhythms
b. is contraindicated in asphyxial arrests
c. should be given without interruption of chest compressions
d. precipitates if mixed with bicarbonate
e. is less effective with poor-quality chest compressions.

Question 16

Absolute contraindications to thrombolysis include:

a. previous haemorrhagic stroke
b. previous major surgery within 6 months
c. aortic dissection
d. CNS neoplasm
e. gastrointestinal bleed within the past month.

Question 17

With regard to drug calculations:

a. 1 ml 1:1000 adrenaline = 10 ml 1% adrenaline
b. 10 ml 50% dextrose = 5 g dextrose
c. 5 ml 0.5% bupivacaine = 2.5 mg bupivacaine
d. 1000 ml 0.9% saline = 9 g saline
e. 10 ml 1% lignocaine = 100 mg.

Question 18

Mouth-to-mouth ventilation without a protective barrier has resulted in transmission of the following pathogens to the rescuer:

a. hepatitis A
b. hepatitis B
c. hepatitis C
d. HIV
e. cytomegalovirus (CMV).

Question 19

Therapeutic hypothermia following cardiac arrest:

a. is recommended for all patients following resuscitation from a VF arrest
b. must be commenced within 30 min of return of spontaneous circulation
c. may induce VF in patients if the core temperature falls below 32°C
d. is most accurately monitored using rectal temperature
e. should be continued for 24–48 h.

Question 20

Techniques of inducing therapeutic hypothermia include:

a. tepid sponging
b. administration of iced (4°C) 0.9% saline IV at 10 ml/kg
c. ice packs
d. cooling mattress
e. bladder irrigation using iced saline (4°C).

Photograph questions

Question 1

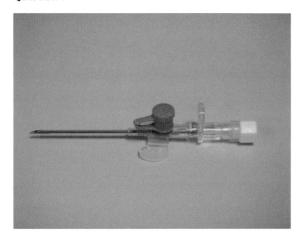

a. What is the relationship between flow rate and cannula diameter?
b. What volume of fluid should be used to flush resuscitation drugs given by this device in an adult?
c. Where is the optimal site for gaining IV access during cardiac arrest?

Question 2

This patient is undergoing emergency thoracotomy for a stab wound to the right ventricle.

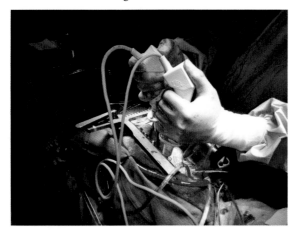

a. What procedure is being performed in this picture?
b. What is the optimal energy for an adult patient?
c. What additional procedure can the paddles be used for?

Question 3

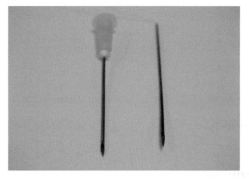

a. What diseases may be transmitted by needlestick injury?
b. What are the risk factors for needlestick injury?
c. What are the risk factors for disease transmission?

Question 4

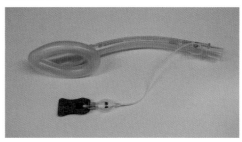

a. What is this?
b. What are the advantages compared with tracheal intubation?
c. What are the disadvantages compared with tracheal intubation?

Question 5

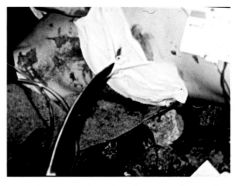

a. What procedure has been performed
b. What are the indications?
c. What are the complications?

Diagnostic questions

Question 1

This CXR is that of a 27-year-old male who has been admitted to the emergency department with sudden onset of severe breathlessness. What is the cause?

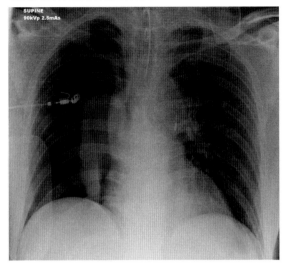

Question 2

A patient is admitted unconscious, with the following arterial blood gases:

pH	7.21
Pao_2	9.1 kPa
$Paco_2$	8.8 kPa
HCO_3^-	25 mmol/l

a. What do these blood gases show?
b. What is the likely cause?

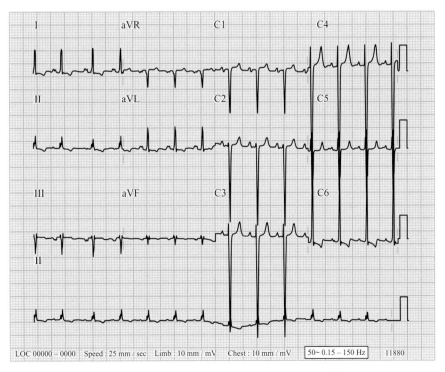

Question 3

This patient has had several episodes of syncope. What is the cause of their collapse suggested by the ECG?

Question 4

A patient is brought into the emergency
department with a penetrating chest injury.

- What does the CXR (right) show?
- What sex is the patient?

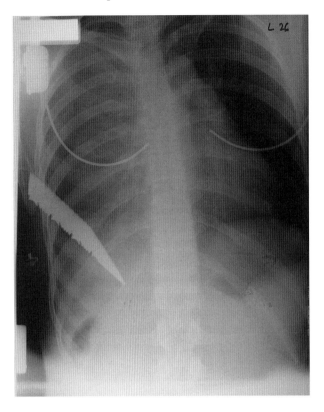

Question 5

What mode is the pacemaker set to in this patient?

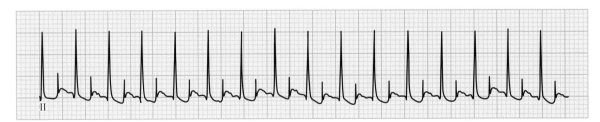

Short answer questions

Question 1

Discuss the use of Intralipid in the management of cardiac arrest caused by local anaesthetic toxicity.

Question 2

What effect does PEEP have on haemodynamics during cardiac massage?

Question 3

Draw the algorithm for paediatric BLS.

Question 4

How will an automatic implantable cardioverter–defibrillator (AICD) behave during a VF arrest?

Question 5

A patient pulled unconscious from a swimming pool has a weak, slow pulse and is unconscious. What are the possible diagnoses?

MCQ answers

Answer 1

a. **False**. Shortened PR interval.
b. **True**.
c. **True**.
d. **False**. Increased R wave amplitude.
e. **True**.

Answer 2

a. **True**.
b. **False**.
c. **False**.
d. **True**.
e. **False**. P waves are not present in atrial fibrillation.

Answer 3

a. **True**.
b. **False**. Infusing a litre of fluid at 40°C to an adult with a core temperature of 28°C increases temperature by only 0.3°C.
c. **False**. Fluids should be administered at 40°C.
d. **True**. Extracorporeal rewarming is the most effective method and provides cardiovascular support at the same time.
e. **True**.

Answer 4

a. **False**. The sinoatrial node stimulates the atrioventricular node during normal sinus rhythm.
b. **True**.
c. **True**. This prevents conduction of rapid atrial impulses to the ventricle, e.g. atrial fibrillation/flutter.
d. **True**.
e. **False**. The ventricular lead of a pacemaker is usually placed to directly stimulate the right ventricular apex.

Answer 5

a. **True**.
b. **False**. The negative intrathoracic pressure increases venous return.
c. **False**. The valve should only be used in conjunction with cardiac arrest.
d. **True**.
e. **False**. The ITD is contraindicated for traumatic cardiac arrest.

Answer 6

a. **True**.
b. **True**.
c. **False**. Mattresses result in movement of the patient, which limits the compression depth achieved during manual CPR.
d. **False**. There is no evidence that chest compressions performed on a beating heart cause arrhythmias.
e. **True**.

Answer 7

a. **True**.
b. **True**. Myocardial perfusion occurs during both the compression and the decompression phase of external chest compressions, although flow is greatest during the decompression phase.
c. **True**.
d. **False**. Coronary perfusion declines with time owing to a gradual reduction in vascular tone and an increase in right atrial pressure.
e. **True**.

Answer 8

a. **True**.
b. **False**. The risk of stroke increases seven-fold for untreated AF.
c. **True**.
d. **False**. May respond to synchronized cardioversion. Unsynchronized shocks risk inducing VF if delivered during the T wave.
e. **True**.

Answer 9

a. **True**.
b. **True**.
c. **False**. Because of the polymorphic nature of torsades, a synchronized cardioversion is not possible, and the patient may require an unsynchronized shock.
d. **True**.
e. **True**.

Answer 10

a. **True**.
b. **True**.
c. **False**. Although biphasic waveforms are more effective at termination of VF/ventricular flutter for any given energy level, no studies have

demonstrated superior survival to hospital discharge.

d. **True.**

e. **True.** Studies comparing monophasic and biphasic waveforms for cardioversion have demonstrated more severe burns (skin erythema) when using monophasic defibrillators.

Answer 11

a. **False.** Increase in survival of 2- to 3-fold has been documented in several studies.

b. **False.** Bystander CPR rates vary considerably but are usually no more than about 30%.

c. **True.** This is thought to be because relatives are too overcome with the situation to perform effectively.

d. **True.**

e. **False.**

Answer 12

a. **True.** Heroin is diacetylmorphine.

b. **True.**

c. **True.**

d. **False.** Morphine is less lipid soluble than diamorphine so it is absorbed more slowly across mucous membranes than diamorphine.

e. **False.** Methadone is a full μ-opioid agonist.

Answer 13

a. **True.** Although earlier models were powered by air or O_2.

b. **False.** The compression cup does not provide a seal on the patient's chest; therefore, the decompression phase is passive.

c. **True.**

d. **True.**

e. **True.**

Answer 14

a. **False.**

b. **True.**

c. **False.**

d. **False.**

e. **True.**

Answer 15

a. **False.** Adrenaline is given as soon as vascular access is achieved for non-shockable rhythms.

b. **False.** Asphyxial arrests are managed using the standard algorithm.

c. **True.**

d. **False.**

e. **True.**

Answer 16

a. **True.**

b. **False.** Previous major surgery within 3 weeks.

c. **True.**

d. **True.**

e. **True.**

Answer 17

a. **False.** 1 ml 1:1000 adrenaline $= 1$ mg adrenaline, but as 1% adrenaline is 10 mg/ml, 10 ml $= 100$ mg.

b. **True.** 50% dextrose $= 500$ mg/ml. Therefore, 10 ml $= 5000$ mg $= 5$ g.

c. **False.** 0.5% bupivacaine $= 5$ mg/ml. Therefore, 5 ml $= 25$ mg.

d. **True.** 0.9% saline $= 9$ mg/ml. Therefore, 1000 ml $= 9000$ mg $= 9$ g.

e. **True.** 1% lignocaine $= 10$ mg/ml. Therefore 10 ml $= 100$ mg.

Answer 18

a. **False.**

b. **False.**

c. **False.**

d. **True.**

e. **False.**

Answer 19

a. **False.** Only patients who remain unresponsive.

b. **False.** The optimal timing is not known.

c. **False.** A core temperature below 28°C is generally considered the threshold at which VF may be induced.

d. **False.** Rectal temperature is usually about 0.5–1.0°C above true core temperature.

e. **False.** Current guidelines recommend a period of 12–24 h, although the optimal period is not known.

Answer 20

a. **False.** Tepid sponging is only used for reducing a fever, usually in children.

b. **False.** 30 ml/kg.

c. **True.**

d. **True.**

e. **True.**

Photograph answers

Answer 1

a. The relation between cannula diameter and flow rate is given by the Hagen–Poiseuille equation, which states that for laminar flow, flow rate ($\dot{Q}$) is given by

$$\dot{Q} = \frac{P\pi r^4}{8\eta L}$$

where P is pressure, r is the radius of the tube, L is its length and η is viscosity.

b. Drugs injected peripherally must be followed by a flush of at least 20 ml of fluid to facilitate drug delivery to the central circulation.

c. Compared with a peripheral cannula, peak drug concentrations are higher and time to reach the central circulation is shorter when drugs are injected into a central venous catheter. However, peripheral venous cannulation is usually quicker and easier than central venous cannulation and is associated with fewer complications.

Answer 2

a. Internal cardioversion (the patient is being defibrillated during open heart surgery).

b. For biphasic shocks, 20 J is the optimal energy level to achieve first-shock success and should be used in an arrest situation.

c. Internal paddles can be used to perform cardiac compressions while charging the defibrillator and delivering the shock, which may improve shock success.

Answer 3

a. Hepatitis A, hepatitis B, hepatitis C, HIV. More rarely, the following diseases have also been documented:
  - blastomycosis
  - brucellosis
  - cryptococcosis
  - diphtheria
  - cutaneous gonorrhoea
  - herpes infection
  - malaria
  - mycobacteriosis
  - mycoplasma caviae

  - Rocky Mountain spotted fever
  - sporotrichosis
  - *Staphylococcus aureus* infection
  - *Streptococcus pyogenes* infection
  - syphilis
  - toxoplasmosis
  - tuberculosis.

b. Risk factors for injury:
  - inexperienced staff
  - attempting to resheath the needle
  - emergency situations.

c. Risk factors for disease transmission:
  - patient with known transmissible disease
  - hollow bore needle
  - deep injury
  - visible blood on the device which caused the injury.

Answer 4

a. Laryngeal mask airway.

b. Advantages:
  - easier and quicker to insert
  - less training needed
  - less skill fade as the insertion procedure is less complex
  - does not require direct visualization of the vocal cords.

c. Disadvantages:
  - does not protect from aspiration (although it does appear to provide some protection, particularly from pharyngeal debris)
  - does not allow such high airway pressures as air will escape from around the cuff at high ventilation pressures
  - may be more easily dislodged compared with a tracheal tube.

Answer 5

a. Chest drain (tube) insertion.

b. Large simple pneumothorax, tension, pneumothorax, haemothorax.

c. Complications:
  - vascular damage (intercostal vessels, mediastinal vessels)
  - organ damage (heart, liver)
  - surgical emphysema.

Diagnostic answers

Answer 1

The CXR shows a right tension pneumothorax. The right lung has collapsed and is visible as a dense peri-hilar mass. The pneumothorax is beginning to tension, as shown by the severely collapsed lung and a slight shift of the mediastinum to the left.

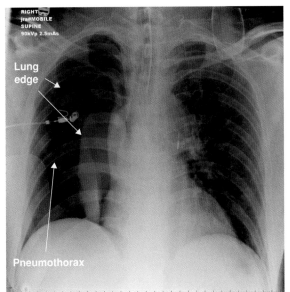

Answer 2

a. These blood gases show a marked acute respiratory acidosis.
b. Airway obstruction caused by impaired level of consciousness, resulting in hypoventilation.

Answer 3

The ECG shows left ventricular hypertrophy (LVH) with strain (ST depression) in the lateral leads. The ECG changes of LVH (Framingham criteria; Levy D *et al. Circulation*,1990; 81:815–820) are:

- R avl > 11 mm, R V4–6 > 25 mm
- S V1–3 > 25 mm, S V1 or V2 +
- R V5 or V6 > 35 mm, R I + S III > 25 mm.
  - These ECG changes are typical of aortic stenosis, which may cause syncope (fainting spells) in 10–20% of patients.

Answer 4

The CXR shows a knife embedded in the right chest. A large right haemothorax is seen. The underwired bra suggests that the patient is female.

Answer 5

The rhythm strip below shows regular pacing spikes (arrowed in the strip here) followed by a QRS complex.

- There is no pacing spike associated with the QRS complex (although there is first-degree heart block). This is, therefore, an atrially paced mode: either AAI or AOO. (It is not possible to tell whether it is a mode inhibited when the intrinsic rate rises above the set threshold (AAI) or a fixed rate mode (AOO).)

Short answers

Answer 1

Intralipid 20% has been shown to reverse local anaesthetic-induced cardiac arrest in animal models, and case reports suggest that it may also be of benefit in the treatment of human toxicity. Patients with cardiac arrest caused by local anaesthetic toxicity may benefit from treatment with IV 20% lipid emulsion in addition to standard ALS. Treatment comprises an initial IV bolus of Intralipid 20% 1.5 ml/kg while CPR is continued. This should be followed by an IV infusion at 0.25 ml/kg per min. Two further boluses of lipid may be given at 5 min intervals while the infusion continues until the patient is stable or has received a maximum of 12 ml/kg body weight lipid emulsion. (For further details, see www.lipidrescue.org, http://www.aagbi.org/sites/default/files/la_toxicity_2010_0.pdf.)

Answer 2

Use of PEEP reduces venous return to the heart by decreasing the pressure gradient between blood in the vena cava and the thoracic cavity, which is normally at a lower pressure. It also acts to cause direct compression of the heart, reducing venous filling and subsequent stroke volume. Therefore, PEEP reduces cardiac output generated during cardiac massage and so reduces subsequent blood pressure.

Answer 4

On sensing a shockable rhythm, an AICD will usually discharge approximately 40 J through an internal pacing wire embedded in the right ventricle. The AICD device will discharge no more than eight times before deactivating, even if a shockable rhythm persists.

Answer 5

The commonest cause of unconsciousness in this circumstance is drowning. However, in this patient, the slow pulse suggests that a high spinal cord lesion is a distinct possibility, most likely caused by a cervical spine injury when diving into the pool.

Answer 3

2010 Resuscitation Guidelines

Resuscitation Council (UK)

Paediatric Basic Life Support
(Healthcare professionals with a duty to respond)

UNRESPONSIVE?

↓

Shout for help

↓

Open airway

↓

NOT BREATHING NORMALLY?

↓

5 rescue breaths

↓

NO SIGNS OF LIFE?

↓

15 chest compressions

↓

2 rescue breaths
15 compressions

Call resuscitation team

Reproduced with permission from the Resuscitation Council (UK).

Multiple choice questions

Question 1

A child is brought in to the emergency department having swallowed some unknown tablets and suffers a VF cardiac arrest. The following tablets may be possible causes:

a. β-blockers
b. tricyclic antidepressants
c. angiotensin-converting enzyme (ACE) inhibitors
d. antiepileptics
e. aspirin.

Question 2

The following are associated with anaphylactic or anaphylactoid reactions:

a. packed red cells
b. platelets
c. fresh frozen plasma
d. colloids
e. crystalloids.

Question 3

The following drugs may cause respiratory depression:

a. doxapram
b. fentanyl
c. atropine
d. diazepam
e. oxygen.

Question 4

With regard to pulse oximetry:

a. cyanide poisoning may cause over-reading
b. carboxyhaemoglobinaemia (HbCO) may cause under-reading
c. movement artefacts cause over-reading
d. hypothermia may cause under-reading
e. ear lobe readings are approximately 1% higher than those obtained on the finger.

Question 5

With regard to IV fluids:

a. 'normal saline' is the same as 0.9% sodium chloride
b. colloids include Hartmann's solution and 5% dextrose
c. 5% dextrose is hypotonic
d. a 70 kg adult requires approximately 3000 ml maintenance fluid /24 h
e. 1000 ml Hartmann's solution contains 10 mmol potassium chloride.

Question 6

With regard to defibrillation safety:

a. current guidelines recommend removing free flowing O_2 at least 1 m away from the patient
b. a ventilator circuit should be disconnected prior to defibrillation
c. 24% O_2 doubles the rate of combustion
d. it is safe for the rescuer's hands to remain in contact with the patient's chest during defibrillation
e. self-adhesive defibrillation pads may reduce the likelihood of arcing compared with defibrillation paddles.

Question 7

Naloxone:

a. has a short half-life, which may result in a recurrence of opioid side effects that it is being used to treat
b. does not interfere with postoperative opioid analgesia
c. may cause fitting when given to opioid-dependent patients
d. when used to treat opioid overdose, should be administered as an initial adult dose of 0.4 mg IV
e. cannot be administered IO.

Question 8

Causes of pulseless electrical activity include:

a. myocardial stunning following defibrillation
b. hyperkalaemia
c. hypothermia
d. hyperthermia
e. hypoglycaemia.

Question 9

Causes of a long QTc interval include:

a. amiodarone
b. lignocaine
c. subarachnoid haemorrhage
d. hypercalcaemia
e. myocardial ischaemia.

Question 10

Drowning:

a. is commonest in children
b. is more common in men than women
c. usually results in cardiac arrest from cooling rather than hypoxaemia
d. often results in vomiting during resuscitation attempts
e. is rarely associated with VF.

Question 11

Causes of hypokalaemia include:

a. chronic constipation
b. diuretics
c. Addison's disease
d. metabolic alkalosis
e. magnesium depletion.

Question 12

Malignant hyperthermia:

a. may be triggered by high-flow O_2 in susceptible individuals
b. may be clinically similar to amphetamine-induced hyperthermia
c. may respond to early administration of rectal dantrolene
d. causing cardiac arrest should be treated using the same techniques as for standard cardiac arrest
e. causes a metabolic acidosis, which may already be severe prior to the cardiac arrest occurring.

Question 13

Acute severe asthma:

a. may respond to Heliox (helium/O_2).
b. when treated with steroids, may result in hypokalaemia
c. when treated with β-agonists, may result in hypokalaemia
d. when associated with a raised $Paco_2$, requires the patient to be intubated
e. may require higher defibrillation energy levels for successful cardioversion.

Question 14

Resuscitative thoracotomy for cardiac arrest:

a. is likely to be more successful for blunt rather than penetrating trauma
b. is unlikely to be successful for unwitnessed cardiac arrest
c. is likely to be less successful for patients with multiple rather than single penetrating injuries
d. should only be performed after tracheal intubation
e. improves survival by facilitating direct intracardiac adrenaline administration.

Question 15

Dopamine:

a. when given as an infusion, may cross the blood–brain barrier to cause nausea and vomiting
b. is broken down by dopamine β-hydroxylase to form noradrenaline
c. in doses from 10 to 20 μg/kg per min are considered 'renal' doses
d. acts as an agonist at β_1-adrenoceptors, resulting in positive inotropic and chronotropic effects
e. acts as an agonist at α_1-adrenoceptors to increase systemic vascular resistance.

Question 16

The following are examples of supraglottic airways:

a. laryngeal mask airway (LMA)
b. i-gel
c. Combitube
d. LMA Supreme
e. tracheostomy.

Question 17

With regard to chest compression depth in children:

a. the chest can be compressed to one-half of the resting anterior–posterior chest diameter without causing damage to intrathoracic organs
b. unlike in adults, good-quality CPR in children is rarely associated with rib fractures
c. it is often too deep
d. in infants, one-third of the chest diameter is approximately 4 cm
e. in children, one-third of the chest diameter is approximately 5 cm.

Question 18

When calculating paediatric drug doses:

a. age-based methods are more accurate than length-based methods in the estimation of body weight
b. in non-obese paediatric patients, initial resuscitation drug doses should be based on actual body weight
c. in obese patients, the initial doses of resuscitation drugs should be based on the ideal body weight
d. doses should be doubled if given by the IO route
e. pre-filled syringes are likely to reduce drug errors.

Question 19

With regard to a pulse check in infants:

a. laypersons are unable to perform an accurate pulse check in infants within 10 s
b. healthcare providers are unable to perform an accurate pulse check in infants within 10 s
c. healthcare professionals perceive a pulse when it is non-existent 5–10% of the time
d. the average time for healthcare providers to detect an actual pulse is approximately 15 s
e. the average time for healthcare providers to confirm the absence of a pulse is approximately 30 s.

Question 20

Heparin:

a. binds to anti-thrombin III, which subsequently inactivates thrombin
b. in its low-molecular-weight form (e.g. Enoxaparin) has anti-factor Xa activity rather than anti-thrombin (IIa) activity
c. slowly breaks down clots that have already formed
d. should be reversed with vitamin K
e. may cause heparin-induced thrombocytopenia (HIT) through the formation of abnormal antibodies that activate platelets.

Photograph questions

Question 1

Core temperature (T1) is being monitored in a patient who is ventilated and sedated on the intensive care unit, 24 h following resuscitation from a cardiac arrest (T2 is peripheral temperature).

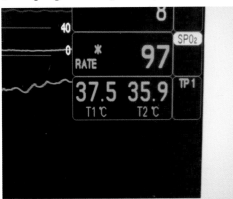

a. Why may this patient be pyrexial?
b. What is the effect of pyrexia on long-term CNS function?
c. What cooling options can be considered?

Question 2

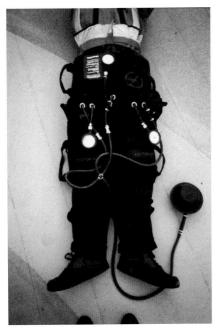

a. What device is fitted to this patient?
b. What is the proposed mechanism of action?
c. Why are these devices now used infrequently?

Question 3

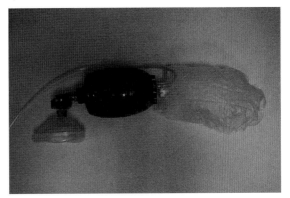

a. How should this circuit be managed during defibrillation?
b. Why does O_2 increase the risk of fire?
c. What resuscitation device may significantly increase ambient O_2 levels during resuscitation?

Question 4

A normal CXR is shown.

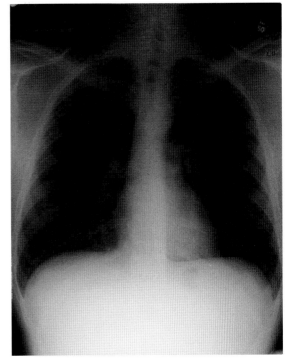

a. How is a normal inspiratory volume assessed on a CXR?
b. What is the cardiothoracic ratio?
c. What chambers of the heart are visible along the edges of the cardiac silhouette?

Question 5

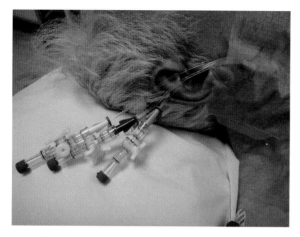

a. What is this?
b. How should this be checked after insertion?
c. The patient suffers a haemodynamic collapse
   during insertion. What are the possible causes?

Diagnostic questions

Question 1

This capnograph trace is recorded during a resuscitation attempt in an intubated patient. What does it indicate?

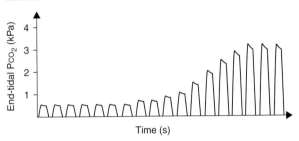

Question 2

A previously well 49-year-old patient presents with sudden onset chest pain and breathlessness with a blood pressure of 82/35 mmHg. Arterial blood gas analysis on air shows the following:

pH	7.29
Pao_2	6.7 kPa
$Paco_2$	3.5 kPa
$HCO_3{}^-$	19 mmol/l
base excess	−5.2 mmol/l

a. What do these indicate?
b. What is the likely diagnosis?
c. What is the differential diagnosis?

Question 3

This patient has suffered a sudden haemodynamic collapse. Their ECG below is shown

a. What does the ECG show?
b. What is the immediate treatment?
c. What type of cardiac surgery procedure is prone to this arrhythmia?

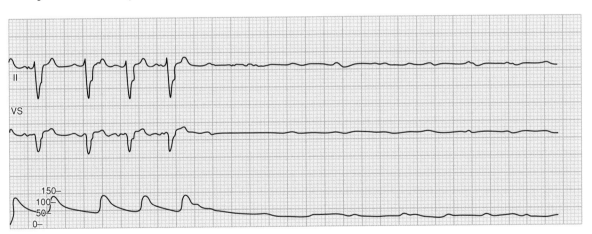

Question 4

What abnormalities are shown in the ECG below?

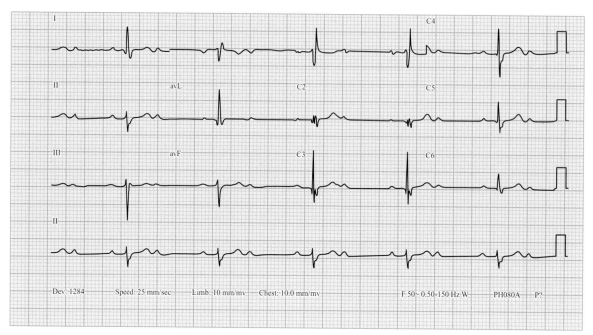

Question 5

A 62 kg, 28-year-old male diabetic presents to the emergency department with Kussmaul breathing and a GCS of 11. Arterial blood gas analysis on room air showed the following result:

pH	7.05
Pao_2	12.2 kPa
$Paco_2$	1.6 kPa
HCO_3^-	4 mmol/l
glucose	18.4 mmol/l

a. What do they indicate?
b. What is the immediate treatment?

Short answer questions

Question 1

What are the causes of respiratory alkalosis following resuscitation from cardiac arrest?

Question 2

In what position should defibrillation electrodes be placed in a patient who has a permanent pacemaker implanted in their right infraclavicular area?

Question 3

Draw a normal end-tidal CO_2 waveform and label the following:

- baseline
- expiratory upstroke
- expiratory plateau
- end-tidal CO_2 value
- beginning of expiration
- end of expiration.

Question 4

Draw the algorithm for adult BLS.

Question 5

A patient suffers a sudden cardiac arrest during the third trimester of pregnancy.

a. What are the most likely causes?
b. Why does delivery of the baby improve cardiac output during CPR?
c. What changes are needed in defibrillation energy for pregnant women at term?

MCQ answers

Answer 1

a. False.
b. True.
c. False.
d. False.
e. False.

Answer 2

a. True.
b. True.
c. True.
d. True.
e. False.

Answer 3

a. False.
b. True.
c. False.
d. True.
e. **True.** In patients with chronic obstructive pulmonary disease, the respiratory centre is driven more by O_2 than CO_2 levels in the blood (hypoxic drive). Excessive O_2 may, therefore, cause respiratory depression in these patients.

Answer 4

a. **False.** Cyanide poisoning may give a high reading because of reduced O_2 extraction from arterial blood; the actual reading is correct.
b. **False.** HbCO may cause over-reading as it has similar absorption of red light as oxyhaemoglobin.
c. **False.** Movement artefacts may cause under-reading.
d. **True.** Hypothermia causes peripheral vasoconstriction and a poor-quality pulse oximetry waveform, which may cause under-reading.
e. **False.** There is no difference.

Answer 5

a. True.
b. True.
c. False.
d. True.
e. **False.** 1000 ml Hartmann's solution contains 5 mmol potassium chloride.

Answer 6

a. True.
b. False.
c. True.
d. False.
e. True.

Answer 7

a. True.
b. False.
c. True.
d. True.
e. True.

Answer 8

a. **True.** May occur in up to 60% of patients following defibrillation.
b. **True.** Hyperkalaemia slows myocardial electrical conduction and depresses myocardial contractility.
c. **True.** Hypothermia causes decreased spontaneous depolarization of pacemaker cells, bradydysrrhythmias and decreased cardiac output.
d. False.
e. True.

Answer 9

a. True.
b. False.
c. True.
d. **False.** Hypocalcaemia causes a prolonged QTc.
e. True.

Answer 10

a. True.
b. **True.** (With the exception of suicide.)
c. **False.** Drowning usually causes hypoxaemic cardiac arrest. Cardiac arrest from rapid cooling only occurs in the most extreme of environmental conditions.
d. **True.** As many as 85% of patients will vomit during BLS.
e. True.

Answer 11

a. **False**. Diarrhoea results in gastrointestinal loss of potassium.
b. **True**.
c. **False**. Addison's disease (adrenal insufficiency) causes hyperkalaemia through impaired aldosterone secretion.
d. **True**.
e. **True**.

Answer 12

a. **False**. Malignant hyperthermia is a life-threatening genetic sensitivity of skeletal muscle, triggered by specific drugs including volatile anaesthetics and depolarizing neuromuscular-blocking drugs.
b. **True**. Other drugs such as MDMA (3,4-methylenedioxymethamphetamine (Ecstasy)) and amphetamines may mimic malignant hyperthermia.
c. **False**. Dantrolene may be effective when given IV.
d. **True**.
e. **True**.

Answer 13

a. **False**. Meta-analysis of four clinical trials failed to demonstrate any benefit from the use of Heliox (mixture of helium and O_2, usually 80:20 or 70:30) in patients with acute severe asthma (Ho A *et al. Chest*, 2003;123:882–890).
b. **True**.
c. **True**.
d. **False**. The overall condition of the patient should be assessed.
e. **True**. Dynamic hyperinflation increases transthoracic impedance, and higher energy levels may be indicated if the initial shocks fail.

Answer 14

a. **False**. Survivors from thoracotomy for blunt trauma are unusual. Most survivors come from patients with penetrating chest injuries.
b. **True**.
c. **True**.
d. **False**. Tracheal intubation performed in order to ventilate the patient is of little benefit without blood flow to the lungs.
e. **False**. There is no evidence that intracardiac adrenaline administration is any more effective than the standard IV route.

Answer 15

a. **False**. Dopamine does not cross the blood–brain barrier.
b. **True**.
c. **False**. Doses from 2 to 5 µg/kg per min are considered 'renal' doses.
d. **True**.
e. **True**.

Answer 16

a. **True**.
b. **True**.
c. **False**. The Combitube does not sit entirely above the glottis and is, therefore, not considered a supraglottic airway (although is classified as such by some authors).
d. **True**.
e. **False**.

(See Miller DM. *Anesth Analg*, 2004;99:1553–1559.)

Answer 17

a. **False**. The chest can be compressed to one-third of the anterior–posterior chest diameter without causing damage to intrathoracic organs; half this chest diameter is associated with organ damage.
b. **True**.
c. **False**. Chest compression depth in children is often too shallow.
d. **True**.
e. **True**.

Answer 18

a. **False**. Length-based methods are more accurate than age-based methods in the estimation of body weight.
b. **True**.
c. **True**. Administration of drug doses based on actual body weight in obese patients may result in drug toxicity.
d. **False**. IO doses are the same as IV doses.
e. **True**.

Answer 19

a. **True.**
b. **True.**
c. **False.** Healthcare professionals perceive a pulse when it is non-existent 14–24% of the time.
d. **True.**
e. **True.**

(See Tibballs J, Russell P *Resuscitation*, 2009;80:61–64.)

Answer 20

a. **True.**
b. **True.**
c. **False.** Heparin does not act on clots that have already formed.
d. **False.** The action of heparin should be reversed with fresh frozen plasma or its derivatives.
e. **True.**

Photograph answers

Answer 1

a. Post-cardiac arrest syndrome (inflammatory phase following resuscitation from cardiac arrest), sepsis, aspiration pneumonia.

b. Several studies have shown an association between post-cardiac arrest pyrexia and poor neurological outcome.

c. External methods:
  - ice packs
  - cooling blankets/mattresses
  - intranasal cooling device.

  Internal methods:
  - cold IV saline (4 ml/kg IV)
  - intravascular cooling catheter.

Answer 2

a. 'Military anti-shock trousers' or 'pneumatic anti-shock garment'.

b. When inflated, the garment is thought to increase systemic vascular resistance in the legs and decrease blood flow to the legs (increasing distribution of blood to the rest of the body), thus squeezing blood out of the lower body.

c. The evidence for their benefit is limited and they may actually increase blood loss by increasing blood pressure. There are also cases of catastrophic haemodynamic collapse following their removal in hypovolaemic patients.

Answer 3

a. This bag-valve-mask is a common breathing circuit used during resuscitation. Current guidelines recommend that the ventilation bag is left connected to the tracheal tube or supraglottic airway device. Alternatively, it is acceptable to disconnect the bag-valve device and remove it at least 1 m from the patient's chest during defibrillation.

b. Fire requires a triad of components: O_2, fuel and heat. Oxygen, therefore, supports combustion. 24% O_2 doubles the rate of combustion; 30% O_2 increases the rate 10-fold.

c. Any device delivering O_2 during the resuscitation attempt: all open-circuit airway devices (oxygen masks, disconnected bag-valve devices) and the LUCAS device when powered by O_2 (discharges O_2 at approximately 100 l/min).

Answer 4

a. Seven to eight anterior ribs should be visible at the lung edge, with the dome of the hemidiaphragms lying at a level of the 6th anterior rib (right higher than left).

b. The cardiothoracic ratio is the distance from the left lateral border of the heart to the right lateral border (a), expressed as a ratio of the overall distance across the chest (b): (a/b). It is normally less than 0.50 (see figure below).

c. The right border of the heart is the edge of the right atrium. The right ventricle sits anteriorly and, therefore, does not have a border on the posterior–anterior CXR. The inferior and left borders of the heart form the left ventricle.

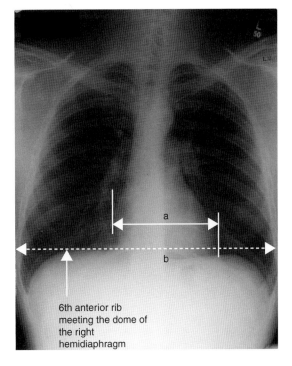

6th anterior rib meeting the dome of the right hemidiaphragm

Answer 5

a. Central venous multiple-lumen catheter.
b. Correct insertion indicated by:
   - auscultation of the chest should show equal air entry on both sides of the chest
   - CXR, performed to ensure appropriate positioning and to exclude any pneumothorax
   - blood should be able to be aspirated freely from all lumens
   - pressure within the lumen of the catheter should be appropriate for the central venous pressure.

c. Potential causes:
   - VF/VT (ventricular fibrillation/tachycardia) from wire
   - tension pneumothorax
   - haemothorax
   - chlorhexidine anaphylaxis (from chlorhexidine coating on the catheter).

Diagnostic answers

Answer 1

This capnograph trace initially shows a low end-tidal CO_2 reading, each peak corresponding to a manual breath. A rapid increase in end-tidal CO_2 is likely to indicate return of spontaneous circulation and is a well-documented and useful marker of this event. A recent study has documented an average increase in end-tidal CO_2 of 13.5 mmHg (1.8 kPa) associated with return of spontaneous circulation (Grmec S *et al. Resuscitation*, 2007;72:404–214).

Answer 2

a. These arterial blood gases show an acute metabolic acidosis with marked hypoxaemia. Hypocapnia results from hyperventilation in an attempt to correct the acidosis.
b. Acute pulmonary embolus.
c. Differential:
   - acute coronary syndromes
   - aortic dissection
   - cardiac tamponade
   - pneumonia
   - pneumothorax
   - septicaemia.

Answer 3

a. This ECG shows sinus rhythm progressing to P wave asystole.
b. Initial treatment is ideally dual chamber pacing. In patients connected to pacing leads (internal or external), pacing should be recommenced. If this is not an immediate option, ALS should be commenced; adrenaline may help to restore a rhythm that generates a cardiac output. Ultimately, this patient is likely to require an internal pacing wire (initially temporary).
c. Aortic valve replacement may damage the bundle of His, which runs past the aortic valve. If atrioventricular conduction is interrupted, the patient risks a cessation of ventricular activity, resulting in P wave asystole, as shown here, or complete heart block.

Answer 4

Right bundle branch block, 2:1 block.

Answer 5

a. These arterial blood gases indicate severe metabolic acidosis. The acidosis is partly compensated as shown by the low Pa_{CO_2}. These patients are severely dehydrated and acidotic.
b. Initial therapy consists of rehydration (using 0.9% saline), control of blood glucose and consideration of the use of bicarbonate to assist with the correction of acid–base status.

Short answers

Answer 1

The commonest cause is iatrogenic, resulting from hyperventilation by the rescuer. Other causes include:

- salicylate intoxication (results in a mixed disorder (metabolic acidosis and respiratory alkalosis))
- pneumonia (where a hypoxic drive governs breathing more than CO_2 levels)
- pulmonary embolism
- asthma
- pulmonary oedema
- pregnancy (compensated respiratory alkalosis).

Answer 2

The sternal pad placed in the standard position (below the right clavicle to the right of the sternum) will risk pacemaker and myocardial damage as electrical current may flow through the pacemaker box and down the pacing wire directly into the myocardial tissue. In a patient with a pacing box placed in the right infra-clavicular position, the pads may be placed in any of the following positions:

- apex to apex (biaxillary)
- anterior (left sternal border) to posterior (medial to the left scapula)
- apex to posterior (behind the right shoulder).

Answer 3

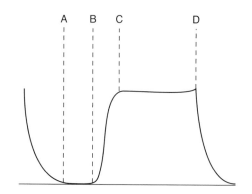

A–B: baseline
B–C: expiratory upstroke
C–D: expiratory plateau
D: end-tidal CO_2 value
D–A: beginning of expiration
B: end of expiration.

Answer 4

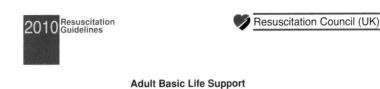

Adult Basic Life Support

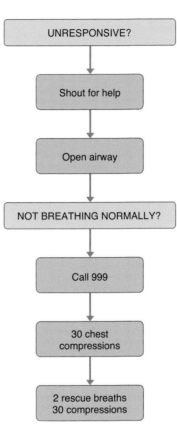

Reproduced with permission from the Resuscitation Council (UK).

Answer 5

a. Likely causes:
  - cardiac disease
  - pulmonary embolism
  - hypertensive disorders of pregnancy: sepsis, haemorrhage, amniotic-fluid embolism.
b. Relief of maternal inferior vena cava compression, which otherwise limits venous return to the heart.
c. There is no change in transthoracic impedance during pregnancy, suggesting that standard shock energies for defibrillation should be used in pregnant patients.

Multiple choice questions

Question 1

The following drugs may cause hyperkalaemia:

a. ACE inhibitors
b. non-steroidal anti-inflammatory drugs
c. spironolactone
d. furosemide
e. amiodarone.

Question 2

The intra-aortic balloon pump (IABP):

a. when optimally positioned, sits between the right subclavian artery and renal arteries
b. uses helium to inflate the endovascular balloon
c. inflates during diastole
d. increases coronary perfusion pressure
e. increases myocardial O_2 consumption.

Question 3

Causes of ECG ST depression include:

a. right bundle branch block
b. left bundle branch block
c. myocardial ischaemia
d. ventricular hypertrophy
e. digoxin effect.

Question 4

The commonest chamber of the heart injured by a stab wound to the chest is:

a. right atrium
b. right ventricle
c. left atrium
d. left ventricle
e. all these in equal frequency.

Question 5

In the management of anaphylaxis:

a. relatively large volumes of IV fluid may be required
b. if a patient is receiving IV colloid at the time of onset of anaphylaxis, it may be a cause of the anaphylaxis and should be stopped
c. steroids may lessen the severity of anaphylaxis
d. glucagon can be useful to treat anaphylaxis in a patient taking a β-blocker
e. the initial blood sample for mast cell tryptase (to help to confirm a diagnosis of anaphylaxis) should be taken as soon as possible after the onset of anaphylaxis.

Question 6

The Purkinje fibres of the heart:

a. are located in the inner ventricular walls of the heart, just beneath the endocardium
b. have no pacemaker capability
c. are specialized to rapidly conduct impulses
d. run into the ventricular tissue from the atrioventricular node
e. divide into left and right-sided conducting pathways.

Question 7

Oxygen:

a. should be reduced following return of spontaneous circulation to achieve a SaO_2 94–98%
b. should not be administered to a neonate during the initial stages of resuscitation
c. is present in Entonox at 30%
d. utilization is inhibited by cyanide, which inhibits mitochondrial cytochrome oxidase to block oxidative metabolism
e. delivered from a cylinder is colder than the ambient temperature.

Question 8

Ventricular tachycardia (VT):

a. when pulsatile, should be treated using the same algorithm as for VF
b. may be monomorphic or polymorphic
c. when polymorphic in nature, is less likely to be associated with a cardiac output than monomorphic VT
d. may be terminated by overdrive pacing
e. requires lower energy levels to cardiovert than does VF.

Question 9

Atropine:

a. blocks the effect of the vagus nerve at both the sinoatrial and atrioventricular nodes
b. side effects include excess salivation and polyuria
c. may cause an acute confusional state, particularly in the elderly
d. is given as a 1 mg IV bolus for bradycardia in adults
e. has a maximum recommended dose of 3 mg IV.

Question 10

Commotio cordis:

a. results from a direct blow to the precordium
b. may be induced by a precordial thump performed during a resuscitation attempt
c. results only if injury occurs during a vulnerable phase of the ECG, during the descending phase of the T wave
d. is not a risk when wearing a sports chest protector
e. has VF as its initial arrhythmia.

Question 11

With regard to coronary artery anatomy:

a. the right and left coronary arteries originate from the aortic root
b. the anatomic definition of dominance is the artery that gives off supply to the sinoatrial (SA) node
c. in 70% of people, the left coronary artery is dominant
d. the left coronary artery divides to form the left anterior descending and circumflex arteries
e. the right coronary artery supplies 25–35% of the left ventricle.

Question 12

Synchronized defibrillation shocks are indicated for the following arrhythmias:

a. atrial fibrillation
b. atrial flutter
c. unstable ventricular tachycardia
d. VF
e. torsades de pointes.

Question 13

Loss of an end-tidal CO_2 trace in a ventilated patient may be caused by:

a. therapeutic hypothermia
b. tracheal tube obstruction
c. ventilator disconnection
d. endobronchial intubation
e. hypoxic gas mixture.

Question 14

With regard to drug administration:

a. drugs given through a peripheral cannula should be followed by a 20 ml flush with 5% dextrose
b. a central venous cannula is preferable to a peripheral cannula if both are available to use
c. IO access should be attempted if central venous cannulation fails
d. administration via the tracheal tube should only be used as a last resort in adults during cardiac arrest
e. subcutaneous administration of adrenaline is appropriate for treatment of an anaphylactic reaction.

Question 15

Blast injuries:

a. are classified as primary, secondary, tertiary and quaternary
b. are more likely to injure solid organs than air-filled viscera
c. primary blast injuries are generally characterized by the absence of external injuries
d. in a confined space are more severe than in open air
e. traumatic brain injury is the most common cause of death among people who initially survive an explosion.

Question 16

β-adrenoceptor blockers:

a. may worsen symptoms by impairing left ventricular function
b. are used for rate control of atrial fibrillation
c. are used for rate control of ventricular tachycardia
d. may be of use to manage cocaine overdose
e. include esmolol, which has the shortest half-life.

Question 17

Signs of raised intracranial pressure include:

a. hypotension
b. tachycardia
c. pupillary constriction
d. Cheyne–Stokes respiration
e. hyperventilation.

Question 18

The precordial thump:

a. has a success rate for VF of approximately 40%
b. is more likely to be successful for pulseless ventricular tachycardia than VF
c. should only be used at a witnessed, monitored arrest when a defibrillator is not present
d. can be repeated in quick succession up to three times
e. may convert a perfusing to a non-perfusing rhythm.

Question 19

Complications of internal jugular vein cannulation include:

a. pneumothorax
b. tracheal puncture
c. air embolus
d. carotid artery puncture
e. atrial arrhythmias.

Question 20

Amiodarone:

a. is indicated after a third shock has been given if the patient remains in a shockable rhythm
b. is administered at the same time as a further dose of adrenaline
c. causes hypotension partly through non-competitive β-blockade
d. causes hypotension partly through action of the solvent rather than the drug itself
e. causes hypotension partly through a negative inotropic effect.

Photograph questions

Question 1

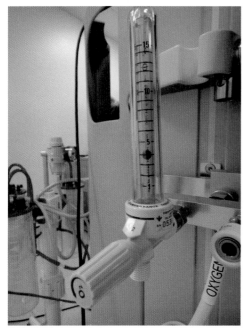

a. What is the name of this device?
b. What gas is delivered by the device?
c. What is the flow rate of the gas being delivered in this photograph?

Question 2

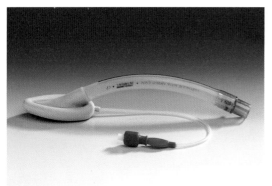

a. What is this airway and to what class of airway does this airway belong?
b. List the advantages of this airway compared to tracheal intubation.
c. List the disadvantages of this airway compared to tracheal intubation.

Question 3

This has been removed from a patient's pulmonary artery.

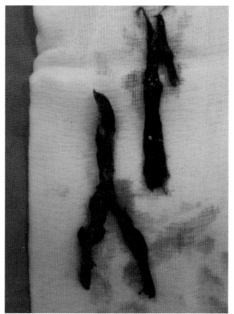

a. What is it?
b. What are the indications for surgical removal?

Question 4

List the electrolyte content of this litre of Hartmann's solution.

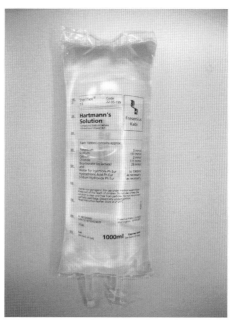

Question 5

This is a cross-section of the larynx. Label structures
A, B, C and D.

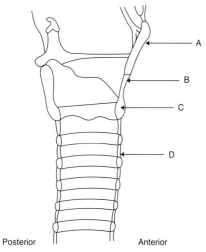

Posterior   Anterior

Diagnostic questions

Question 1

The following femoral blood gases are taken from a patient following return of spontaneous circulation, with blood pressure 101/56 mmHg, pulse 121, sinus rhythm and arterial haemoglobin saturation (SpO_2) 95% on 40% O_2:

pH	7.32
PaO_2	4.5 kPa
$PaCO_2$	7.4 kPa
HCO_3^-	26 mmol/l
SaO_2	75%

What is the likely diagnosis?

Question 2

This is a pressure trace of an intra-aortic balloon pump (IABP). Describe the events occurring at A, B, C and D.

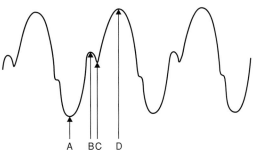

Question 3

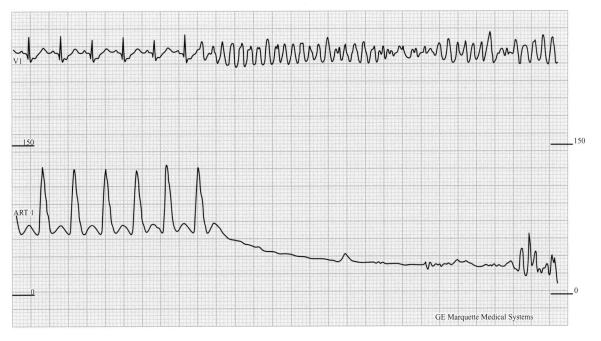

a. What does this recording show?
b. What is the immediate treatment?

Question 4

This is the waveform capnograph tracing from a ventilated patient who has suffered a respiratory arrest. What is the likely cause of their respiratory deterioration?

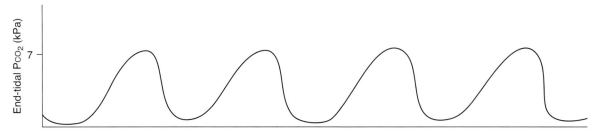

Question 5

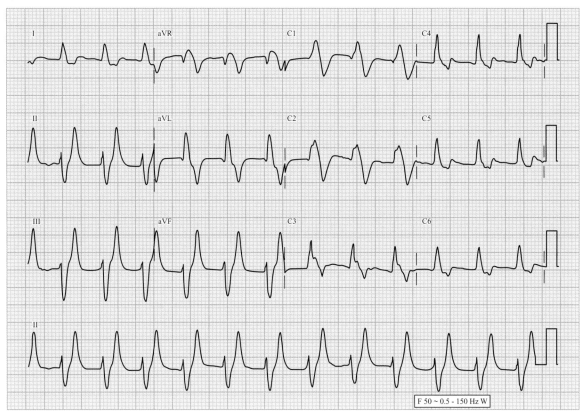

a. List the abnormalities in this ECG.
b. What metabolic disturbance might have caused these changes?

Short answer questions

Question 1

Draw a picture of the heart showing the four main chambers, aorta and pulmonary artery. Add the normal values for systolic and diastolic pressures in the right and left ventricles, aorta and pulmonary artery. Add the normal mean pressure in the right and left atria.

Question 2

A patient is brought in to the emergency department in an acute confusional state with a sinus tachycardia of 145/min and a core temperature of 41.1°C. List drugs that are associated with a hyperthermic response.

Question 3

Draw the O_2 dissociation curve, labelling P_{50}. List factors that shift the curve to the right and left.

Question 4

List the normal values (pH, P_{CO_2}, P_{O_2}, HCO_3^-, base exess) for arterial and venous blood gases in a healthy patient.

Question 5

A patient who suffers a cardiac arrest has been taking the following drugs; which ones will affect the resuscitation attempt?

a. β-blockers
b. clopidogrel
c. monoamine oxidase inhibitors.

MCQ answers

Answer 1

a. **True.**
b. **True.**
c. **True.**
d. **False.**
e. **False.**

Answer 2

a. **False.** Sits between the left subclavian and renal arteries.
b. **True.**
c. **True.**
d. **True.**
e. **False.** Decreases myocardial O_2 consumption by decreasing afterload and, therefore, myocardial workload.

Answer 3

a. **False.**
b. **True.**
c. **True.**
d. **True.**
e. **True.**

Answer 4

a. **False.**
b. **True.**
c. **False.**
d. **False.**
e. **False.** The right ventricle presents the largest area and is involved in 45% of penetrating myocardial injuries. The left ventricle is involved in 35%, right atrium in 10% and left atrium in 5%.

Answer 5

a. **True.** Leakage of large volumes of fluid from the patient's circulation combined with vasodilation may result in significant hypovolaemia.
b. **True.**
c. **True.** Although the evidence for their benefit is lacking.
d. **True.**
e. **True.**

Answer 6

a. **True.**
b. **False.** Are capable of acting as the pacemaker if the sinoatrial and atrioventricular nodes fail.
c. **True.** Purkinje cells contain numerous sodium ion channels and mitochondria, but fewer myofibrils than the surrounding muscle tissue.
d. **False.** The atrioventricular node sends impulses to the bundle of His, which then connects to the Purkinje fibres.
e. **True.**

Answer 7

a. **True.**
b. **True.** Supplemental O_2 is only indicated if the neonate remains hypoxic.
c. **False.** Entonox contains 50% O_2 and 50% nitrous oxide (N_2O).
d. **True.**
e. **True.** Expansion of a gas as it emerges from a pressurized cylinder results in a drop in its temperature. (The ratio between the pressure–volume product and the temperature of a system remains constant: $P \propto 1/T$, where P is the pressure and T the absolute temperature.)

Answer 8

a. **False.** Only when non-pulsatile is the VF treatment algorithm appropriate for the treatment of VT.
b. **True.** Monomorphic VT means that the appearance of all the beats match each other in each lead of a surface ECG; polymorphic VT has beat-to-beat variations in morphology.
c. **True.** Polymorphic VT is usually torsades de pointes, which is associated with a loss in cardiac output.
d. **True.**
e. **False.** The same energy level protocols as for VF are indicated for VT.

Answer 9

a. **True.**
b. **False.** Side effects include blurred vision, dry mouth and urinary retention.
c. **True.**
d. **False.** The recommended dose is 500 μg IV.
e. **True.**

Answer 10

a. **True.**
b. **False.** A precordial thump is performed because the patient is already suffering a ventricular arrhythmia.

c. **False.** Results only if injury occurs during the ascending phase of the T wave.

d. **False.** People wearing chest protectors make up 20% of cases.

e. **True.**

Answer 11

a. **True.**

b. **False.** The anatomic definition of dominance is the artery which gives off supply to the atrioventricular (AV) node: the AV nodal artery.

c. **False.**

d. **True.**

e. **False.** In 70% of people, the right coronary artery is dominant.

Answer 12

a. **True.**

b. **True.**

c. **False.**

d. **False.**

e. **False.**

Answer 13

a. **False.**

b. **True.**

c. **True.**

d. **False.**

e. **False.**

Answer 14

a. **False.** Drugs given through a peripheral cannula should be followed by a 20 ml flush with 0.9% saline.

b. **True.** Because central venous drug administration results in quicker delivery of drugs to the myocardium.

c. **False.** Intraosseous access should be attempted if perpheral cannulation cannot be gained quickly.

d. **False.** Absorption of drugs by this route is poor and the fluid causes impaired gas exchange. It should not be used.

e. **True.**

Answer 15

a. **True.** Primary injuries are from blast/shock waves; secondary, from bomb fragments; tertiary from blast wind throwing victims against solid objects; and quaternary, burns and rush injuries.

b. **False.** Lungs and air-filled viscera are particularly susceptible to shock waves.

c. **True.**

d. **True.**

e. **False.** Blast lung is the most common cause of death among people who initially survive an explosion.

Answer 16

a. **True.**

b. **True.**

c. **False.**

d. **True.** Cocaine causes intense sympathetic stimulation.

e. **True.** The half-life of esmolol is approximately 5 min.

Answer 17

a. **False.** Hypertension (increased systolic blood pressure).

b. **False.** Bradycardia.

c. **False.** Pupillary dilatation.

d. **True.** An abnormal breathing with cyclical increases and decreases in respiratory rate and depth.

e. **True.**

Answer 18

a. **False.** Reported success rates for VF are <5%.

b. **True.**

c. **True.**

d. **False.**

e. **True.**

(See Pellis T, Kohl P. *Br Med Bull*, 2010;93:161–177.)

Answer 19

a. **True.**

b. **True.**

c. **True.**

d. **True.**

e. **True.**

Answer 20

a. **True.**

b. **True.**

c. **False.** Causes hypotension through non-competitive α-blockade.

d. **True.**

e. **True.**

Photograph answers

Answer 1

a. Rotameter.
b. Oxygen (labelled on the control knob).
c. 4 l/min (the rate is measured from the centre of the ball).

Answer 2

a. This is a laryngeal mask airway, which is a supraglottic airway.
b. Advantages
   - Easier to insert as it does not require direct visualization of the larynx (Can be used as a rescue device when tracheal intubation fails).
   - Requires less training and operator experience for successful insertion.
   - Slower skill fade in LMA insertion, compared with tracheal intubation.
   - Quicker to insert than a tracheal tube.
   - Causes less increase in intracranial pressure compared with tracheal intubation.
   - Results in less movement of the cervical spine during insertion.
   - Avoids unrecognized oesophageal intubation.
c. Disadvantages
   - Does not allow suctioning of the tracheal and upper airway.
   - Less effective route for drug administration (although tracheal drug administration during cardiac arrest is no longer recommended as drug absorption is so poor).
   - More likely to become dislodged during patient movement, compared with a correctly secured tracheal tube.
   - Limited peak airway pressure can be achieved, because air leaks from around the cuff at airway pressures in excess of 15–20 cm H_2O.
   - Gastric insufflation may occur if the cuff is over-inflated.

Answer 3

a. This is a blood clot that has caused an acute pulmonary embolus. It is a classic saddle embolus that sits astride the junction of the right and left pulmonary artery.
b. A large pulmonary embolus may cause a cardiac arrest (hypotension progressing to pulseless electrical activity). Although use of thrombolytic drugs may be effective in some patients, surgical removal may be more effective in peri-arrest/ arrest as it immediately removes the obstruction rather than waiting up to 90 min for the thrombolytic drug to dissolve the clot sufficiently for circulation to be restored.

Answer 4

Contents:

Na^+	131 mmol/l
K^+	5 mmol/l
Ca^{2+}	2 mmol/l
Lactate	29 mmol/l

Answer 5

Structures:

A: thyroid cartilage
B: cricothyroid membrane
C: cricoid cartilage
D: trachea.

Diagnostic answers

Answer 1

These blood gases are inconsistent with the patient's physiological status and are likely to be an accidental venous sample; a low PaO_2 and high $PaCO_2$ with SaO_2 considerably lower than that recorded by pulse oximetry suggests that this is likely. A further sample should be analysed.

Answer 2

Events:

A: end of diastole and beginning of systole
B: end of systole
C: beginning of IABP inflation (at dichrotic notch) as aortic valve closes
D: beginning of IABP deflation.

Answer 3

a. This ECG shows a patient in sinus rhythm developing VF. The arterial pressure trace (lower line) shows a concomitant loss in pulsatile arterial pressure.
b. Immediate treatment is defibrillation (150–200 J biphasic shock; 360 J monophasic shock). If this is witnessed and the patient is already connected to a defibrillator, it is acceptable to give three quick stacked shocks (as necessary) before commencing chest compressions.

Answer 4

This waveform, often described as a 'shark fin' in appearance, is typical of patients with bronchospasm. It differs from the normal square wave in the delayed rise of the expiratory phase resulting from the limited expiratory airflow. This patient had suffered a respiratory arrest from acute asthma.

Answer 5

a. This ECG shows:
   - reduction of the size of the P wave
   - peaked T waves
   - widening of the QRS complex.
b. These changes are typical of hyperkalaemia (this patient's potassium was 8.6 mmol/l), which should be treated.

79

Short answers

Answer 1

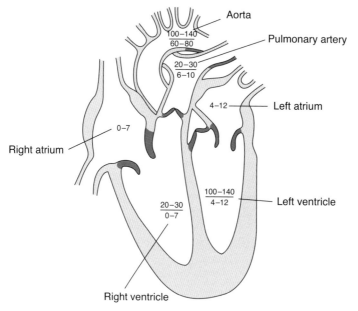

Answer 2

Hyperthermia is associated with:

- haloperidol
- chlorpromazine
- dothiepin
- levodopa
- metoclopramide
- lithium
- monoamine oxidase inhibitors
- cocaine
- tricyclic antidepressants
- atropine
- glycopyrrolate
- droperidol
- ketamine
- Ecstasy
- alcohol withdrawal.

Answer 3

Graph of percentage O_2 saturation (So_2) versus oxygen partial pressure Po_2.

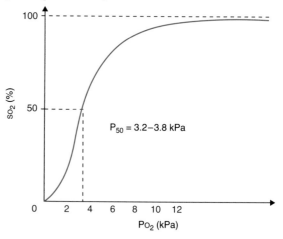

- P_{50} is the oxygen partial pressure at which haemoglobin is 50% saturated
- **Left shift** (increased affinity of haemoglobin for O_2) is caused by:
  - hypothermia
  - hypocapnia
  - alkalosis
  - increased 2,3-DPG (2,3-diphosphoglycerate).
- **Right shift** (decreased affinity of haemoglobin for O_2) is caused by:
  - hyperthermia
  - hypercapnia
  - acidosis
  - decreased 2,3-DPG.

Answer 4

	Arterial	Venous
pH	7.35–7.45	7.32–7.42
P_{CO_2}	4.7–6.0 kPa (35–45 mmHg)	5.9–6.4 kPa (44–48 mmHg)
P_{O_2}	9.3–13.3 kPa (80–110 mmHg)	5.4 kPa (40 mmHg)
HCO_3^- (mmol/l)	22–26	21–22
Base excess (mmol/l)	−2 to 2	−2 to 2

Answer 5

a. • Stimulation of β_1-adrenoceptors increases force and rate of myocardial contractility
   • Stimulation of β_2-adrenoceptors induces smooth muscle relaxation.

β-blockers block β-adrenoceptors in the heart, bronchi and peripheral vasculature. β-blockers, therefore, act to slow force and rate of myocardial contraction and may worsen bronchospasm. Patients taking β-blockers who suffer a cardiac arrest may require greater doses of adrenaline (although 1 mg adrenaline every second cycle is still recommended). Peri-arrest bradycardia is often refractory to anticholinergic drugs (atropine/glycopyrrolate) and may require sympathomimetics (adrenaline, dopamine, etc.) to increase heart rate.

b. Clopidogrel is an oral antiplatelet drug prescribed to patients at risk of coronary artery thrombosis. It acts by binding to an ADP receptor on the platelet surface to inhibit platelet aggregation and fibrin cross-linking. The incidence of haemorrhage in these patients is 0.1–0.4% (cerebral) and 2.0% (gastrointestinal). Risks are increased in patients also taking aspirin. Patients suffering a cardiac arrest who have been taking these drugs may also be at increased risk of localized bruising from external chest compression and of haemorrhagic complications (cardiac tamponade, intracerebral bleed).

c. Monoamine oxidase inhibitors inhibit monoamine oxidase to cause an accumulation of amine neurotransmitters (adrenaline, noradrenaline, dopamine) resulting in an enhancement of their effect. The effect of adrenaline is, therefore, enhanced and prolonged. It has been suggested that the adrenaline dose should be reduced by 75%. Noradrenaline and dopamine, if administered, should also be used with caution, ideally titrated to effect using invasive arterial monitoring.

Multiple choice questions

Question 1

With regard to compression:ventilation during CPR:

a. a ratio of 30:2 is recommended for lay rescuers
b. a ratio of 15:2 is recommended for paediatric resuscitation by trained rescuers
c. compressions should be delivered before ventilation in adults
d. compressions should be delivered before ventilation in children
e. compression-only CPR is an acceptable alternative for bystander BLS.

Question 2

Benzodiazepine overdose:

a. may cause hypertension
b. may cause respiratory arrest
c. may require higher than normal adrenaline doses during CPR
d. should not be reversed with flumazenil in patients with a history of epilepsy
e. in patients with co-ingestion of tricyclic antidepressants flumazenil is contraindicated.

Question 3

In the treatment of severe acute asthma:

a. nebulized adrenaline may be effective if nebulized salbutamol does not improve the patient's condition
b. steroids given IV are preferable to oral steroids as the onset of action is quicker
c. nebulized magnesium sulphate (250 mmol/l in a volume of 2.5–5 ml) may improve pulmonary function
d. nebulized ipratropium bromide (0.5 mg) may be of benefit in patients who do not respond to β-agonists
e. patients with asthma are at increased risk of anaphylaxis.

Question 4

Magnesium:

a. when indicated, is given as a 1 mg IV bolus
b. may be repeated after 10–15 min
c. is indicated for refractory VF
d. improves the contractile response of the stunned myocardium
e. may cause hypotension when given as a rapid bolus.

Question 5

Causes of pulseless electrical activity include:

a. hypovolaemia
b. cardiac tamponade
c. tension pneumothorax
d. paracetamol overdose
e. pulmonary embolus.

Question 6

In-hospital cardiac arrests:

a. are preceded by signs of physiological deterioration in as few as 30% of patients
b. are associated with successful resuscitation to hospital discharge in approximately 50% of cases
c. present most commonly as non-shockable arrhythmias
d. that are called in error are associated with a 30% eventual mortality in this group of patients
e. should always trigger a crash call even if the patient has a 'Do Not Attempt Resuscitation' order.

Question 7

With regard to electrical safety during defibrillation:

a. biphasic defibrillators discharge voltages up to 2800 V
b. biphasic defibrillators discharge currents up to 30 A
c. gloves provide safety from inadvertent shock
d. self-adhesive electrodes are safer than manual paddles
e. leakage current during defibrillation may damage manual chest compression devices.

Question 8

Digoxin toxicity:

a. is exacerbated by hypokalaemia
b. causes blurred vision, with visual disturbances and yellow–green visual halos
c. causes ST elevation in ECG
d. is not usually responsive to haemodialysis
e. can be treated with potassium supplements.

Question 9

With regard to respiratory effort:

a. the intercostal muscles and diaphragm are the main muscle groups
b. the diaphragm is supplied by the vagus nerve
c. diaphragmatic innervation arises from cervical nerves C3, C4, and C5
d. hypoventilation may occur secondary to multiple sclerosis and Guillain–Barré syndrome
e. hyperphosphataemia may cause severe respiratory muscle weakness.

Question 10

Causes of complete heart block include:

a. mitral valve surgery
b. infective endocarditis
c. ischaemic heart disease
d. calcium channel blocker overdose
e. digoxin overdose.

Question 11

Calcium is indicated for pulseless electrical activity arrests caused by:

a. hyperkalaemia
b. overdose of calcium channel-blocking drugs
c. hypocalcaemia
d. hypomagnesaemia
e. metabolic alkalosis.

Question 12

The definition of an acute coronary syndrome includes:

a. stable angina
b. unstable angina
c. Non-ST elevation acute myocardial infarction
d. ST elevation acute myocardial infarction
e. pericarditis.

Question 13

Mouth-to-mouth ventilation without a protective barrier has resulted in transmission of the following pathogens to the rescuer:

a. *Salmonella*
b. *Staphylococcus aureus*
c. meningococcal meningitis
d. *Shigella*
e. cutaneous tuberculosis.

Question 14

With regard to drug efficacy:

a. adrenaline increases the rate of return of spontaneous circulation but has not been shown to increase survival to hospital discharge
b. amiodarone increases the rate of return of spontaneous circulation compared with lignocaine
c. atropine increases the rate of return of spontaneous circulation but has not been shown to increase survival to hospital discharge
d. colloids have been shown to be more effective than crystalloids in achieving return of spontaneous circulation following hypovolaemic cardiac arrest
e. bicarbonate increases the rate of return of spontaneous circulation, but has not been shown to increase survival to hospital discharge.

Question 15

Dobutamine:

a. is a structural analogue of dopamine
b. causes vasodilation through α-antagonist activity
c. is a β_1-adrenergic agonist, with weak activity at β_2-adrenceptors
d. is a racemic mixture
e. may worsen the haemodynamic status of patients in atrial fibrillation.

Question 16

Cardiac arrest:

a. presents as VF as the initial rhythm in approximately 60% of cases of out-of-hospital arrest
b. has approximately double the survival rate in patients with a shockable compared with non-shockable rhythm
c. has survival rates that have been gradually improving since the early 2000s
d. occurs in one-third of all people who suffer an out-of-hospital myocardial infarction
e. has an increase in mortality of approximately 10% for each minute's delay in ambulance arrival.

Question 17

With regard to ECG leads:

a. a 3-lead ECG involves leads placed on the right arm, left arm and abdomen/left lower chest wall
b. a 12-lead ECG involves 12 leads placed as for a 3-lead ECG, together with anterior chest leads (V1–V6)
c. lead I is the optimal lead with which to diagnose the rhythm

d. lead V5 is the optimal lead to monitor myocardial ischaemia
e. shivering often causes a poor ECG signal by dislodging an ECG electrode.

Question 18

Waveform capnography:

a. is recommended for routine use in patients intubated at a cardiac arrest
b. when used to verify tracheal tube placement during cardiac arrest, has approximately 80% sensitivity and specificity
c. can provide an indicator of cardiac output if minute ventilation volume is fixed
d. can be used to distinguish asystole from VF
e. will not distinguish between tracheal and endobronchial placement of the tracheal tube tip.

Question 19

Relative contraindications to thrombolysis include:

a. ongoing CPR
b. pregnancy
c. aspirin therapy
d. infective endocarditis
e. active peptic ulcer disease.

Question 20

Cricothyroidotomy:

a. is the same procedure as a tracheostomy
b. involves an incision through the thyroglossal membrane
c. involves the same anatomical pathway as insertion of a 'Minitrach'
d. is indicated for a 'can't ventilate, can't intubate' situation
e. may result in venous bleeding from the incision that is difficult to control.

Photograph questions

Question 1

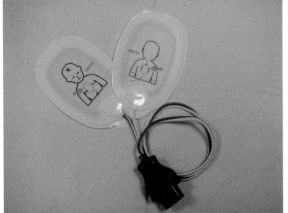

a. What are these?
b. What is the weight limit of children in which these should be used?
c. Where should they be placed anatomically?

Question 2

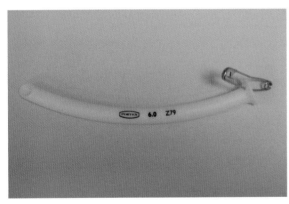

a. What is this?
b. When should it be used?
c. In whom may this be contraindicated?

Question 3

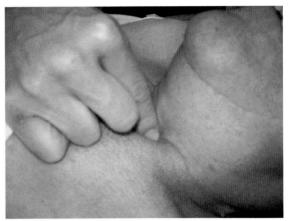

a. What procedure is being performed here?
b. What are the indications for this procedure?
c. How is it correctly performed?

Question 4

Name the heart valves labelled A, B, C, and D.

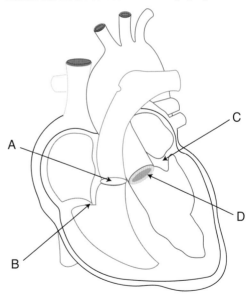

Question 5

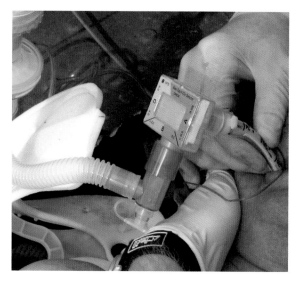

a. What is this device?
b. What colour changes does it go through?
c. What are its limitations?

Diagnostic questions

Question 1

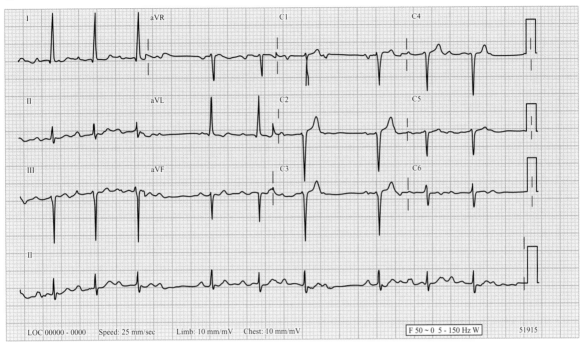

What rhythm is shown in this ECG?

Question 2

A 23-year-old woman with a known psychiatric history has taken an overdose of an unknown drug. She is brought in to the emergency department hyperventilating, confused and vomiting. The arterial blood gas on air is shown below. What is the likely drug?

pH	7.50
Pao_2	17.3 kPa
$Paco_2$	3.9 kPa
HCO_3^-	19 mmol/l

Question 3

A patient is resuscitated from a cardiac arrest. They are subsequently intubated and mechanically ventilated. While waiting for transfer from the emergency department to the intensive care unit, the previously stable capnograph trace shows the following pattern. What event is likely to be occurring?

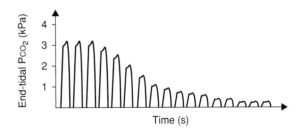

Question 4

The following are O_2 saturations (on air) measured from blood samples withdrawn by cardiac catheter from each respective cardiac chamber of a heart.

right atrium	70%
right ventricle	85%
pulmonary artery	85%
left atrium	100%
left ventricle	100%
aorta	100%

What is the diagnosis?

Question 5

What is the cause of breathlessness in this patient?

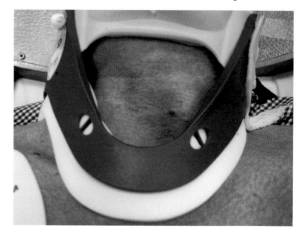

Short answer questions

Question 1

List the physiological changes in the cardiovascular system that occur during pregnancy.

Question 2

What are the National Institute for Clinical Excellence (NICE) guidelines for IV pre-hospital fluid administration? Write a short summary.

Question 3

List the causes of respiratory alkalosis.

Question 4

Draw the algorithm for adult ALS.

Question 5

What additional measures are taken during the resuscitation of a pregnant mother at term?

MCQ answers

Answer 1
a. **True.**
b. **True.**
c. **True.**
d. **False.**
e. **True.**

Answer 2
a. **False.** May cause hypotension.
b. **True.**
c. **False.**
d. **True.** In these patients, flumazenil may trigger seizures.
e. **True.** Flumazenil can be associated with significant toxicity (seizure, arrhythmia, hypotension and withdrawal syndrome) in patients with co-ingestion of proconvulsant medications such as tricyclic antidepressants.

Answer 3
a. **False.** There is no evidence that nebulized adrenaline is any more effective than nebulized salbutamol.
b. **False.** Adminstering steroids IV has not been shown to have an effect any quicker than the oral route, although patients with acute severe asthma may have difficulty in swallowing medication.
c. **True.**
d. **True.**
e. **True.** Patients with asthma have a higher incidence of allergies, and anaphylaxis may be difficult to distinguish from severe life-threatening asthma.

Answer 4
a. **False.** When indicated, is given as a 2 mg IV bolus.
b. **True.**
c. **False.** Is indicated only for arrhythmias associated with hypomagnesaemia (supraventricular tachycardia, ventricular tachycardia) or torsades de pointes.
d. **True.**
e. **True.**

Answer 5
a. **True.**
b. **True.**
c. **True.**
d. **False.**
e. **True.**

Answer 6
a. **False.** Are preceded by signs of physiological deterioration in at least 80% of patients.
b. **False.** Are associated with successful resuscitation to hospital discharge in only 20% of cases.
c. **True.**
d. **True.**
e. **False.** Cardiac arrest calls are not indicated in these patients.

Answer 7
a. **True.**
b. **True.**
c. **True.** However, gloves may breakdown at the voltages seen during defibrillation and are often torn during resuscitation attempts, rendering them ineffective as an electrical barrier.
d. **True.** Manual paddles require the rescuer to lean over the patient during defibrillation, unlike self-adhesive pads, which allow the rescuer to stand clear from the patient.
e. **False.** LUCAS2 and Autopulse devices are safe to use with ongoing defibrillation.

Answer 8
a. **True.** Because digoxin normally competes with K^+ for the same binding site on the Na^+/K^+-ATPase pump.
b. **True.**
c. **False.** ST depression.
d. **True.** Digoxin is not removed by haemodialysis with enough effectiveness to treat toxicity.
e. **True.**

Answer 9

a. **True.**
b. **False.**   Phrenic nerve.
c. **True.**
d. **True.**
e. **False.**   Hypophosphataemia may cause severe respiratory muscle weakness.

Answer 10

a. **False.**   Aortic valve surgery may disrupt the bundle of His and cause complete heart block.
b. **True.**   May be indicative of an aortic root abscess.
c. **True.**
d. **True.**
e. **True.**

Answer 11

a. **True.**
b. **True.**
c. **True.**
d. **False.**
e. **False.**

Answer 12

a. **False.**
b. **True.**
c. **True.**
d. **True.**
e. **False.**

Answer 13

a. **True.**
b. **True.**
c. **True.**
d. **True.**
e. **True.**

Answer 14

a. **True.**
b. **True.**
c. **False.**   Atropine has not been shown to be effective for any arrhythmia associated with cardiac arrest.
d. **False.**
e. **False.**

Answer 15

a. **False.**   It is a structural analogue of isoprenaline.
b. **False.**   Vasodilation results from β_2-agonist activity.
c. **True.**
d. **True.**   The $(+)$ isomer is a potent β_1-agonist and α_1-antagonist. The $(-)$ isomer is an α_1-agonist. The administration of the racemate results in the overall β_1-agonism.
e. **True.**   By causing a marked increase in ventricular rate through an increase in atrioventricular node conduction.

Answer 16

a. **False.**   Presents as VF in approximately 30% of cases of out-of-hospital arrest.
b. **True.**
c. **True.**
d. **True.**
e. **True.**

Answer 17

a. **True.**
b. **False.**   A 12-lead ECG involves four limb leads and six chest leads. The 12 'leads' are a combination of vectors from these 10 leads (I, II, III, aVL, aVR, aVF, V1, V2, V3, V4, V5, V6).
c. **False.**   Lead II is the optimal lead as the P waves are the largest magnitude in this lead.
d. **True.**
e. **False.**   Shivering causes a poor ECG signal through movement artefact and muscle tremor.

Answer 18

a. **True.**
b. **False.**   Both 100% sensitivity and 100% specificity have been documented for identifying correct tracheal tube placement.
c. **True.**
d. **False.**   Both arrhythmias are associated with cessation of cardiac output.
e. **True.**

Answer 19

a. **False.**
b. **True.**
c. **False.**
d. **True.**
e. **True.**

Answer 20

a. **False.** A tracheostomy is usually performed as an elective/urgent procedure, accessing the airway through the trachea itself.
b. **False.** Involves an incision through the cricothyroid membrane.
c. **True.**
d. **True.**
e. **True.**

Photograph answers

Answer 1

a. Paediatric self-adhesives defibrillation pads.
b. Children <10 kg in body weight.
c. The pads are applied in the anterior–lateral position (one below the right clavicle and the other in the left axilla). If the pads are too large and there is a danger of charge arcing across the pads, use the anterior–posterior position. (One pad on the upper back below the left scapula and the other on the front, to the left of the sternum).

Answer 2

a. Nasopharyngeal airway.
b. The nasopharyngeal airway is used as a basic airway adjunct. In patients with an obstructed airway, it can be used instead of, or together with, an oropharyngeal airway. In patients who are semiconscious, a nasopharyngeal airway is better tolerated than an oropharyngeal airway. The nasopharyngeal airway may be life saving in a patient with a clenched jaw, trismus or maxillofacial injuries, when insertion of an oropharyngeal airway is not possible.
c. In patients with a basal skull fracture, there is a small risk of the nasopharyngeal airway penetrating the skull through the cranial vault. If an oropharyngeal airway cannot be inserted and the airway remains obstructed, gentle insertion of a nasopharyngeal airway may be life saving, far outweighing any risks.

Answer 3

a. Cricoid pressure (Sellick manoeuvre).
b. Cricoid pressure is applied in situations where there may be a risk of regurgitation (and subsequent aspiration) of gastric contents. It may cause difficulty with ventilation, obstruct the airway and make tracheal intubation and supraglottic airway insertion more difficult.
c. Traditional teaching is that 44 N of pressure is required to occlude the oesophagus. This is equivalent to the force required to produce pain when 'cricoid pressure' is applied to the bridge of the nose.

Answer 4

Valves are:
A. pulmonary valve
B. tricuspid valve
C. mitral valve
D. aortic valve.

Answer 5

a. Capnometer.
b. The indicator paper contains a pH-sensitive dye that undergoes a colour change in the presence of CO_2. The dye is usually metacresol purple, which changes to yellow in the presence of CO_2.
c. The limitations are:
   - acidic solutions (lidocaine, adrenaline, atropine) will permanently change the colour to yellow if they come in contact with the indicator paper
   - the device will change colour in a cyclical manner for the first few minutes but eventually the colour change becomes less marked
   - the device has a relatively high dead space, limiting its use for paediatric/neonatal patients, but low dead-space devices are available for this age group
   - only gives a very approximate estimate of end-tidal CO_2 value.

Diagnostic answers

Answer 1

Second-degree heart block (Wenkebach/Mobitz type 1). A P wave is blocked from initiating a QRS complex, but the delay increases with each cardiac cycle until a QRS complex fails to be initiated.

Answer 2

These arterial blood gases show a respiratory alkalosis ($Paco_2$ 3.9 kPa) with a compensatory metabolic acidosis (HCO_3^- 19 mmol/l), which is typical of salicylate overdose, 4 to 6 h after the overdose has been taken. Salicylates act directly to stimulate the respiratory centre, which causes the respiratory alkalosis. A reduced bicarbonate level occurs in an attempt to compensate for the alkalosis.

Answer 3

When a patient is ventilated at a fixed minute volume, changes in end-tidal CO_2 are proportionate to pulmonary blood flow and, therefore, cardiac output. The capnograph trace shows a rapid decline in cardiac output, to very low levels, consistent with a further cardiac arrest.

Answer 4

These are all normal values, except for the pulmonary artery and right ventricle, which would both be expected to be about 70%. Unexpectedly high O_2 saturations are, therefore, present in these two areas, suggesting the presence of a shunt. If the shunt was from the left atrium to the right atrium (e.g. atrial septal defect), higher saturations would be expected in the right atrium. These values suggest that oxygenated blood is flowing into the right ventricle (anatomically, this is only possible from the left ventricle via a ventricular septal defect), as higher than normal saturations are present in the right ventricle (but lower than the left ventricle as the shunt is only partial) – a difference that persists as blood flows into the pulmonary artery. These values are, therefore, consistent with a ventricular septal defect with right-to-left shunt.

Answer 5

This patient has fallen from the roof of a garage. His trachea is shown deviated to the left. It is likely that the cause of his breathlessness is a right-sided tension pneumothorax, which has displaced the trachea to the left.

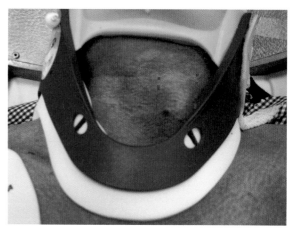

Short answers

Answer 1

Changes in pregnancy include:

- cardiac output increases 30–40% above normal by 32 weeks of gestation
- aortocaval compression reduces cardiac output from 20 weeks onwards
- heart rate increases by 15%, together with an increase in stroke volume of 30%; however, a fall in systemic vascular resistance results in an unchanged blood pressure
- cardiac hypertrophy and dilatation cause ECG changes of left axis deviation, ST depression and flattening/inversion of T wave in lead III
- albumin is diluted, reducing plasma oncotic pressure and predisposing to pulmonary oedema at lower pressures
- progesterone levels are increased in pregnancy and there is reduced protein binding in plasma, which increases myocardial sensitivity to bupivacaine.

Answer 2

The 2004 guidance *Pre-hospital Initiation of Fluid Replacement Therapy in Trauma* (http://egap.evidence. nhs.uk/TA74) covers the management of adults, children and infants with injuries as a result of trauma, with associated blood loss.

- IV fluid should not be administered if a radial pulse can be felt (or, for penetrating torso injuries, if a central pulse can be felt).

- In the absence of a radial pulse (or a central pulse for penetrating torso injuries) in adults and older children, IV fluid should be administered in boluses of no more than 250 ml. The patient should then be reassessed, and the process repeated until a radial pulse (or central pulse for penetrating torso injuries) is palpable.
- The administration of IV fluid should not delay transportation to hospital. Consideration should be given to administration en route to hospital.

Answer 3

Causes of respiratory alkalosis can be divided into:

- **central causes** (direct action via respiratory centre):
  - head injury
  - stroke
  - anxiety-induced hyperventilation
  - salicylate overdose
- **hypoxaemia**:
  - respiratory stimulation (acting via peripheral chemoreceptors)
- **pulmonary causes**:
  - pulmonary embolism
  - pneumonia
  - asthma
  - pulmonary oedema
- **iatrogenic** (act directly on ventilation):
  - excessive minute volume resulting from manual hyperventilation.

Answer 4

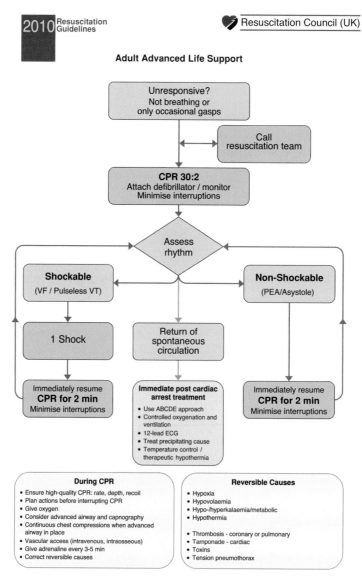

Reproduced with permission from the Resuscitation Council (UK).

Answer 5

Modifications to BLS for a pregnant mother at term are:

- call for expert help immediately
- manually displace the uterus to the left to remove inferior vena cava compression (necessary from 20 weeks of gestation onwards)
- add 15–30° left lateral tilt if this is feasible.

Modifications to ALS are:

- early tracheal intubation with cricoid pressure may reduce the risk of pulmonary aspiration

- tracheal intubation may be more difficult because of maternal airway narrowing from oedema and swelling
- a tracheal tube 0.5–1 mm internal diameter smaller than that used for a non-pregnant woman of similar size may be necessary
- standard shock energies for defibrillation attempts should be used as there is no change in transthoracic impedance during pregnancy; adhesive defibrillator pads are preferable to paddles in pregnancy.

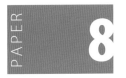
Multiple choice questions

Question 1

ECG changes of hypomagnesaemia include:

a. short PR interval
b. ST depression
c. widened QRS
d. torsades de pointes
e. peaked T waves.

Question 2

Hypothermia may be associated with:

a. the elderly
b. infants
c. drug overdose
d. electrocution
e. anaesthetic induction drugs.

Question 3

With regard to gastric lavage for drug overdose:

a. there is little evidence to support its use
b. should be administered after activated charcoal has been given
c. is contraindicated for hydrocarbons unless the airway is protected
d. is contraindicated for corrosive substances unless the airway is protected
e. is contraindicated for enteric coated drugs.

Question 4

With regard to age groups for specific guidelines:

a. the term newborn refers to a neonate immediately after delivery
b. a neonate is a child within 1 week of age
c. an infant is a child under 1 year of age
d. a child refers to children between 1 year and 8 years

e. adult guidelines are applicable to individuals aged over 18 years.

Question 5

Atropine:

a. is indicated for haemodynamically unstable patients with atrial, nodal or sinus bradycardia
b. is indicated during cardiac arrest with pulseless electrical activity
c. is contraindicated for atrioventricular node block, where it may worsen bradycardia
d. blocks parasympathetic nicotinic acetylcholine receptors
e. precipitates with bicarbonate.

Question 6

In patients with return of spontaneous circulation (ROSC) following resuscitation from cardiac arrest, seizures:

a. occur in 2% of adult patients who achieve ROSC
b. may be masked by neuromuscular-blocking drugs
c. do not affect neurological outcome
d. may result from hypoglycaemia
e. can be controlled by benzodiazepines, phenytoin, sodium valproate, propofol or barbiturates.

Question 7

With regard to adult BLS:

a. on finding an unresponsive patient, two breaths should be given before calling for help
b. if the patient is not breathing normally, they should be placed in the recovery position
c. chest compressions should be given before any rescue breaths
d. it should be continued until the patient shows signs of life
e. fatigue when performing chest compressions occurs after 5 min.

Question 8

Paraquat:

a. is a rat poison
b. may be absorbed by a rescuer giving mouth-to-mouth ventilation
c. poisoning may be lessened by early administration of activated charcoal
d. is selectively accumulated by the lungs
e. lung injury is minimized by early ventilation with 100% O_2.

Question 9

Sudden cardiac death:

a. is most commonly caused by coronary artery disease
b. may also be caused by inherited diseases
c. is not usually associated with prior warning signs such as chest pain, palpitations
d. may present as unexplained drowning
e. should lead to consideration of screening of all family members.

Question 10

Accidental intra-arterial injection:

a. is more of a risk during a resuscitation attempt than in elective treatment
b. usually presents as paraesthesia in conscious patients
c. most commonly involves the radial artery
d. when identified, requires the arterial cannula to be removed immediately
e. treatment includes sympathetic block to improve peripheral vasodilation, anticoagulation to prevent thrombus formation and pain relief.

Question 11

Cyanide:

a. is a common component of residential or industrial fires
b. uncouples mitochondrial oxidative phosphorylation, thus inhibiting cellular respiration
c. inhibition of cellular respiration can be overcome with high-flow O_2 therapy

d. scavengers include hydroxocobalamin, which is used as a cyanide antidote
e. hydroxocobalamin may cause methaemoglobinaemia.

Question 12

When performing internal defibrillation for VF:

a. defibrillation paddles should be placed in contact with the right atrium and left ventricle
b. a synchronized shock is required
c. a 20 J shock achieves more rapid defibrillation and fewer shocks than lower energy levels
d. continuing cardiac compressions using the internal paddles while charging the defibrillator and delivering the shock during the decompression phase of compressions may improve shock success
e. all staff should stand clear of the patient.

Question 13

When treating a patient suffering a cardiac arrest from electrocution:

a. asystole is more likely with a DC shock
b. VF is more likely with an AC shock
c. spinal immobilization should be considered until cervical spine injury can be excluded
d. early tracheal intubation may be needed as airway oedema may progress rapidly
e. rhabdomyolysis may require generous IV fluid resuscitation to minimize renal failure and metabolic acidosis.

Question 14

Nitrates:

a. are converted to nitric oxide to cause smooth muscle vasodilatation
b. are generally contraindicated in patients with a systolic blood pressure <90 mmHg
c. when given as GTN through a puffer are administered as a dose of 100 μg with each puff
d. when given as a transdermal patch, may explode if defibrillation electrodes are in contact with the patch during defibrillation
e. may cause a throbbing headache.

Question 15

In unstable angina:

a. the ECG may be normal
b. the ECG may show evidence of acute ischaemia (e.g. ST depression)
c. the ECG may show non-specific abnormalities (e.g. T wave inversion)
d. troponin levels are, by definition, elevated
e. the patient is at risk of cardiac arrest.

Question 16

In patients with a cocaine overdose:

a. sympathetic block may cause bradycardia and hypotension
b. a cocaine half-life of approximately 1 h can be expected
c. both α- and β-blockers may be required to control hypertension and tachycardia
d. benzodiazepines are contraindicated in treating overdose
e. hyperthermia is common.

Question 17

Mortality from cardiac arrest:

a. usually results from ischaemic myocardial injury
b. is particularly high when cardiac arrest is caused by asphyxia
c. increases by 5% for every minute's delay in ambulance response
d. is reduced by programmes of public-access defibrillation
e. is less for traumatic cardiac arrest than for arrest caused by coronary artery disease.

Question 18

Broad complex tachycardia may be:

a. supraventricular tachycardia with aberrant conduction
b. supraventricular tachycardia with Wolff–Parkinson–White syndrome
c. torsades de pointes
d. nodal tachycardia
e. ventricular tachycardia.

Question 19

Cricoid pressure:

a. is also known as Sellick's manoeuvre
b. requires a backwards force against the cricoid cartilage of 10–20 N
c. applied during bag-valve-mask ventilation reduces gastric insufflation
d. may result in difficulties in supraglottic airway insertion
e. must be released during active vomiting, to reduce the risk of oesophageal rupture.

Question 20

Adult foreign body airway obstruction:

a. is usually a witnessed event
b. is usually caused by laryngospasm induced by food or fluid
c. is defined as mild if the patient can cough
d. if severe, should be treated by giving 5 back blows alternating with 5 abdominal thrusts
e. should be treated with standard BLS if the patient is unconscious.

Photograph questions

Question 1

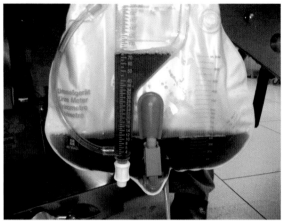

a. Why might this urine be discoloured?
b. What are the possible causes?

Question 2

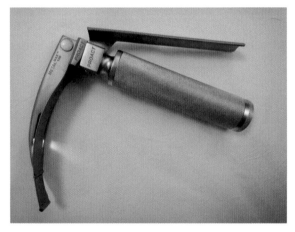

a. What type of laryngoscope is shown in this picture?
b. When might it be used?

Question 3

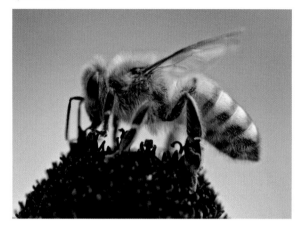

a. What class of insect is this?
b. An adult patient suffers an anaphylactic reaction to a bee sting. What initial symptoms would be expected?
c. The patient has an Epipen. What dose of adrenaline does this device deliver?

Question 4

This is a patient who has been intubated after being rescued from a house fire.

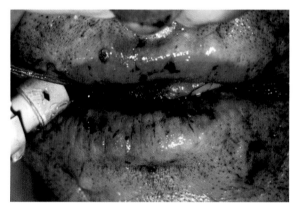

a. What features of the history and examination are suggestive of significant smoke inhalation?
b. How do the levels of carboxyhaemoglobin (HbCO) relate to symptoms?
c. What is the half-life of carboxyhaemoglobin on air and on 100% O_2?

Question 5

This patient has been successfully defibrillated during a cardiac arrest. The defibrillation has resulted in these erythematous skin burns.

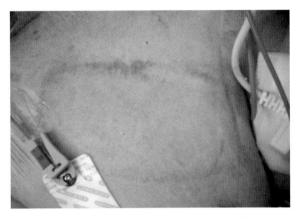

a. Why do the burns only occur at the periphery of the defibrillation electrode?
b. What treatment is appropriate to minimize pain and inflammation from these burns?

Diagnostic questions

Question 1

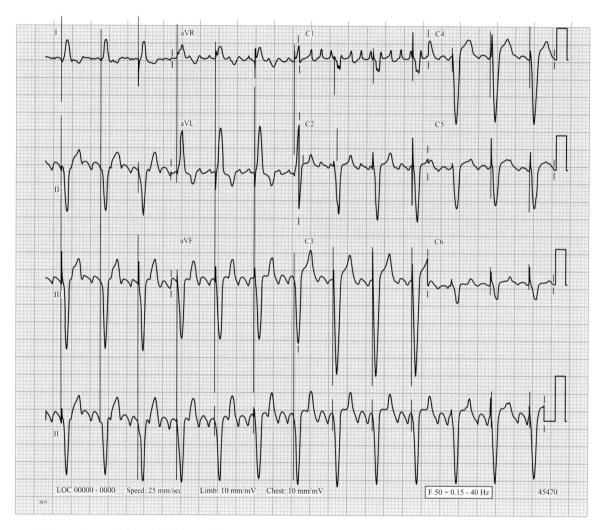

a. What is the underlying rhythm in this ECG?
b. What other abnormalities are present?

Question 2

What abnormality is shown in this waveform capnograph recording?

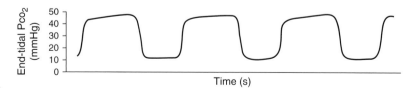

Question 3

What abnormality is shown in this CXR?

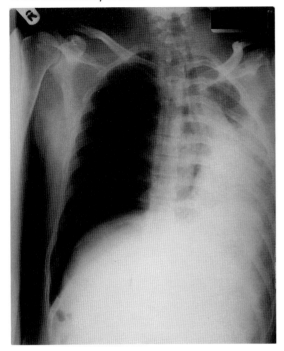

Question 4

A farmer is admitted having collapsed with the following symptoms, having ingested an unknown liquid:

- runny nose, salivation
- chest tightness and difficulty breathing
- constriction of the pupils
- abdominal pain and vomiting.

What type of chemical is most likely to cause these symptoms?

Question 5

a. What rhythm is shown in the ECG below?
b. List common causes.

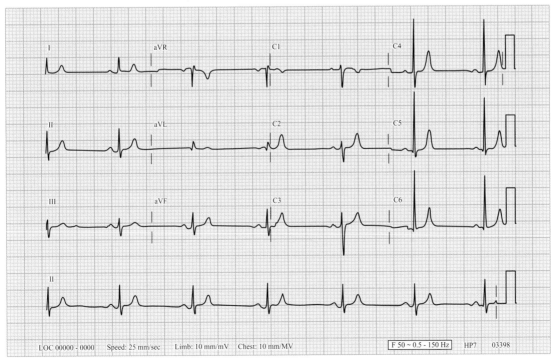

Short answer questions

Question 1

You are called to an intubated patient at a cardiac arrest who is not ventilating when using a self-inflating bag-valve-tracheal tube system.

a. What is the differential diagnosis?
b. How should oesophageal intubation be excluded?

Question 2

Draw a picture of the universal symbol used to indicate the presence of an automatic external defibrillator (AED).

Question 3

List the physiological changes in the respiratory system during pregnancy.

Question 4

Discuss the differences in acid–base state between venous and arterial blood during CPR and the limitations of each in assessing acid–base status.

Question 5

Give the approximate weights (kg) of patients at the following ages:

a. newborn
b. 1 year
c. 2 years
d. 5 years
e. 10 years.

MCQ answers

Answer 1

a. **False.** Prolonged PR interval.
b. **True.**
c. **True.**
d. **True.**
e. **False.** T wave inversion.

Answer 2

a. **True.**
b. **True.**
c. **True.**
d. **False.**
e. **True.** Anaesthetic induction drugs impair responses to thermoregulation.

Answer 3

a. **True.**
b. **False.**
c. **True.**
d. **True.**
e. **False.**

Answer 4

a. **True.**
b. **False.** A neonate is a child within 0 to 4 weeks of age.
c. **True.**
d. **False.** A child refers to children between 1 year and onset of puberty.
e. **False.** Adult guidelines are applicable for individuals from puberty onwards.

Answer 5

a. **True.**
b. **False.** The 2010 resuscitation guidelines removed pulseless electrical activity as an indication for atropine.
c. **False.** Bradycardia associated with atrioventricular node block is an indication for atropine.
d. **False.** Blocks parasympathetic muscarinic acetylcholine receptors.
e. **False.**

Answer 6

a. **False.** Seizures occur in 5–15% of adult patients who achieve ROSC and 10–40% of those who remain comatose.
b. **True.**
c. **False.** Seizures increase cerebral metabolism by up to three-fold and may cause cerebral injury.
d. **True.**
e. **True.**
(See Deakin CD *et al. Resuscitation*, 2010;81: 1305–1352.)

Answer 7

With regard to the sequence in adult BLS:

a. **False.** Help should be called for as soon as the patient is unresponsive. Emergency services should be called before giving any breaths.
b. **False.** Abnormal breathing may be agonal breathing and the patient may require rescue breaths.
c. **True.**
d. **True.**
e. **False.** Fatigue occurs after approximately 2 min.

Answer 8

a. **False.** It is a herbicide.
b. **True.** Mouth-to-mouth ventilation should be avoided in patients with suspected Paraquat poisoning.
c. **True.**
d. **True.**
e. **False.** Lung injury will worsen with 100% O_2. Use 21% O_2 (i.e. air) if possible.

Answer 9

a. **True.**
b. **True.** For example, Brugada syndrome, hypertrophic cardiomyopathy.
c. **False.** Most victims of sudden cardiac death have a history of cardiac disease and warning signs, most commonly chest pain, in the hour before cardiac arrest.
d. **True.**
e. **True.**

Answer 10

a. **True.** Because the cannula is usually inserted in a hurry and the unconscious patient is unable to report symptoms.
b. **False.** Usually presents as local irritation or pain. Paraesthesia usually presents later.
c. **True.** The antecubital fossa and groin are also sites for potential errors because of the proximity of arterial and venous vessels.
d. **False.** Leaving the cannula in situ will allow immediate delivery of multiple medications to the site of injury.
e. **True.**

Answer 11

a. **True.**
b. **True.**
c. **False.** Inhibition of cellular respiration cannot be reversed by adequate O_2 levels.
d. **True.**
e. **True.**

Answer 12

a. **False.** Internal paddles are usually placed across the two ventricles.
b. **False.** Synchronized shocks are not required for VF.
c. **True.**
d. **True.**
e. **True.** Although the low energy levels and direct application over the heart result in minimal risk for anyone in contact with the patient.

Answer 13

a. **True.**
b. **True.**
c. **True.** Secondary injury is common, particularly with high-voltage electrocution.
d. **True.**
e. **True.**

Answer 14

a. **True.**
b. **True.**
c. **False.** A single puff of GTN delivers 400 μg per metered dose.

d. **False.** It is the metal lining of the patch rather than the GTN itself that causes arcing and an explosion.
e. **True.**

Answer 15

a. **True.**
b. **True.**
c. **True.**
d. **False.** Troponin levels may be normal.
e. **True.**

Answer 16

a. **False.** Sympathetic overstimulation can result in agitation, tachycardia, hypertension and coronary vasoconstriction, which causes myocardial ischaemia.
b. **True.**
c. **True.**
d. **False.** Benzodiazepines are indicated to control agitation in cocaine overdose.
e. **True.** Paracetamol and tepid sponging may be inadequate to control the hyperthermia and active measures may be required.

Answer 17

a. **False.** Two-thirds of patients die from neurological injury.
b. **True.**
c. **False.** Increases approximately 7–10% for every minute's delay.
d. **True.** Generally true, providing AEDs are placed in appropriate locations.
e. **False.** Outcome from traumatic cardiac arrest is generally worse.

Answer 18

a. **True.**
b. **True.** The delta wave of Wolff–Parkinson–White syndrome may give the appearance of a widened QRS complex.
c. **True.**
d. **False.**
e. **True.**

Answer 19

a. **True.** (Brian A. Sellick, 1918–1996, Anaesthetist, London, UK.)
b. **False.** Requires 20–40 N.
c. **True.**
d. **True.**
e. **True.**

Answer 20

a. **True.**
b. **False.** Is usually caused by direct obstruction with food.
c. **True.**
d. **True.**
e. **True.**

Photograph answers

Answer 1

a. Urine may be a red/brown colour because of haemolysis or rhabdomyolysis.

b. Causes include:
- **haemolysis:**
  - chronic haemolysis from a faulty heart valve
  - prolonged cardiopulmonary bypass
  - snake venom
- **rhabdomyolysis:**
  - prolonged limb ischaemia
  - severe soft tissue trauma
  - snake venom.

Answer 2

a. This is a McCoy laryngoscope. It is based on the standard Macintosh blade but has a hinged tip that is activated by depression of the associated lever. It enables elevation of the epiglottis to produce a better view of the larynx and vocal cords.

b. It is used in patients where a difficult intubation is anticipated or experienced. It is also used when intubating patients with a suspected cervical spine injury where it enables less flexion of the cervical spine compared with a standard laryngoscope.

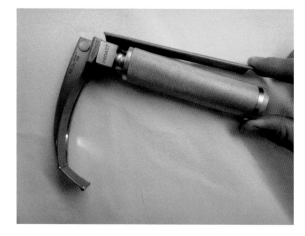

Answer 3

a. This bee is a member of the Hymenoptera family. (*hymen*, membrane; *pteron*, wing).

b. Common symptoms include perioral tingling; swelling of lips, tongue and face; urticarial rash; nausea and vomiting.

c. An Epipen delivers 0.3 mg adrenaline IM. (Epipen Junior delivers 0.15 mg adrenaline IM.)

Answer 4

a. **History** features include:
- patient inside a closed building
- prolonged rescue.

b. **Examination** features include:
- external facial burns
- soot on lips, tongue and/or nostrils
- burn to hard palate
- wheeze
- change in quality of voice
- cough
- high carbon monoxide levels.

b. Symptoms of carbon monoxide poisoning relate to HbCO:

HbCo (%)	Symptoms
0–10	None
10–20	Headache, malaise
30–40	Nausea and vomiting, slowing of mental activity
60–70	Cardiovascular collapse, death.; consider hyperbaric O_2 therapy

c. Half-life on air is 320 min; half-life on 100% O_2 is 80 min.

Answer 5

a. Burns occur in a peripheral pattern because current density is highest at the edges of the defibrillation electrodes.

b. Simple oral analgesia (paracetamol, non-steroidal anti-inflammatory drugs) and topical flamazine (silver sulfadiazine) cream.

Diagnostic answers

Answer 1

a. Atrial flutter.
b. Other abnormality is VVI pacing (pacing spikes can be seen, each of which triggers a QRS complex). (VVI: sensing the ventricle, pacing the ventricle and inhibition by electrical activity sensed in the ventricle.)

Answer 2

A normal capnograph waveform should return to baseline during the inspiratory phase. The waveform shown here does not return to the baseline and this pattern is indicative of rebreathing of exhaled gases in the breathing circuit. As a general principle, the flow rate of the inspiratory gases should be increased until the inspiratory phase of the waveform returns to baseline.

Answer 3

This CXR shows a massive right-sided tension pneumothorax, characterized by:

- collapse of the right lung
- mediastinal shift to the left
- tracheal deviation to the left
- surgical emphysema of the soft tissues (visible in the right axilla).

Answer 4

Organophosphate pesticide poisoning typically causes these symptoms. Signs of organophosphate poisoning include:

- nausea
- headache
- general weakness or tiredness.

This progresses to:

- sweating and salivation
- vomiting and diarrhoea
- pupillary constriction and blurred vision
- muscle tremors
- excessive pulmonary secretions
- epilepsy and loss of consciousness.

Answer 5

a. Sinus bradycardia.
b. Common causes are:
   - drugs: β-blockers, amiodarone, verapamil
   - hypermagnesaemia
   - acute spinal cord injury
   - raised intracranial pressure
   - hypothyroidism.

Short answers

Answer 1

a. Differential diagnosis:
   - aspiration
   - foreign body airway obstruction
   - acute severe asthma/bronchospasm
   - uni/bilateral tension pneumothorax
   - large uni/bilateral haemothorax
   - misplaced tracheal tube (unrecognized oesophageal intubation)
   - obstructed/blocked tracheal tube
   - obstructed/blocked catheter mount
   - faulty ventilation bag.

b. Oesophageal intubation is excluded by clinical assessment and a secondary confirmation technique.

   Clinical assessment:
   - observation of bilateral chest expansion
   - auscultation over both lung fields and epigastrium.

   Secondary **confirmation technique** ensures high levels of sensitivity and specificity:
   - measurement of exhaled CO_2 with end-tidal CO_2 devices:
     - disposable colorimetric devices
     - non-waveform electronic digital devices that have a bar display for CO_2 and/or show a peak value
     - devices with a waveform graphic display
     - **oesophageal detector device:** creates suction at the distal end of the tracheal tube (via a large syringe or releasing a compressed flexible bulb); air is easily aspirated if the tracheal tube is in the trachea but not if it is in the oesophagus
     - **thoracic impedance:** smaller changes in thoracic impedance occur with oesophageal ventilations than with ventilation of the lungs; remains a research tool at present.

Answer 2

Answer 3

Respiratory changes during pregnancy:

- reduction in lung volume resulting from diaphragm elevation; this is compensated by increased transverse and anterior–posterior diameter of the chest allowed by the loosening of ligaments through hormonal effects
- increased minute volume by 40%, increased tidal volume and a 15% increase respiratory rate at term; this results in a respiratory alkalosis that shifts the O_2 dissociation curve to the left. A concomitant increase in P_{50} from 3.5 to 4.0 facilitates O_2 unloading across the placenta
- increased closing capacity, which may exceed the functional residual capacity to cause atelectasis
- increased basal metabolic rate, which increases O_2 consumption.

Answer 4

On cessation of blood flow, arterial blood is rich in O_2 and has normal CO_2 levels (with the exception of cardiac arrest caused by hypoxia or respiratory failure). Static blood in arteries undergoes relatively little gas exchange. Blood in capillaries and end organs continues to undergo gas exchange, with continuing O_2 extraction and build up of CO_2.

- Subsequent cardiac massage moves oxygenated blood into the capillaries and end organs and drives capillary and end organ blood into the venous system. Central venous blood samples taken during cardiac arrest predominantly show a respiratory acidosis (decrease in pH and increase in PCO_2), in contrast to a metabolic acidosis in arterial samples. The difference between central venous PCO_2 and arterial PCO_2 is approximately 5.5 kPa, reflecting the low blood flow in patients undergoing CPR.
- Arterial blood, therefore, does not reflect the marked reduction in tissue pH, and thus arterial blood gases may fail as appropriate guides for acid–base management during CPR. Central (mixed) venous blood most accurately reflects the acid–base state during CPR, particularly the rapid increase in PCO_2.

Answer 5

The traditional formula: weight(kg) $= 2$(age $+ 4$) has been shown to underestimate weight significantly. A more accurate formula is weight(kg) $= 3$(age) $+ 7$. (Luscombe M, Owens B. *Arch Dis Child*, 2007;92:412–415):

a. newborn: 3.5 kg
b. 1 year: 10 kg
c. 2 years: 13 kg
d. 5 years: 22 kg
e. 10 years: 37 kg.

Multiple choice questions

Question 1

Sodium bicarbonate:

a. when indicated, is often given as a bolus of 50 ml 8.4% solution
b. should be considered for cardiac arrest associated with hypokalaemia
c. shifts the O_2 dissociation curve to the right, increasing O_2 delivery to tissues
d. may require an increase in minute ventilation to clear the subsequent generation of CO_2
e. will precipitate if mixed with calcium solutions.

Question 2

Hyperthermia following resuscitation from cardiac arrest:

a. is defined as a core temperature $\geq 37.1°C$
b. is common in these patients
c. is usually a result of sepsis, e.g. aspiration pneumonia
d. can usually be controlled with regular paracetamol
e. may worsen neurological outcome.

Question 3

$\alpha\beta$-adrenoceptor blockers are contraindicated in patients with:

a. chronic constrictive pulmonary disease
b. asthma
c. first-degree heart block
d. second-degree heart block
e. third-degree heart block.

Question 4

The oesophageal detector device:

a. uses a large syringe or bulb attached to the proximal end of the tracheal tube

b. indicates tracheal placement when the syringe plunger cannot be withdrawn or the bulb will not reinflate
c. may be misleading in patients with morbid obesity
d. may be misleading in patients in late pregnancy
e. may be misleading in patients with copious secretions.

Question 5

Aspirin:

a. when administered for acute coronary syndrome, is given as an oral dose of 75 mg
b. may worsen overall morbidity through gastrointestinal bleeding
c. inhibits platelet function
d. inhibits the intrinsic clotting pathway
e. reduces the risk of coronary artery thrombus formation.

Question 6

The internal jugular vein:

a. lies medial to the carotid artery
b. lies at the posterolateral edge of the trachea
c. runs with the phrenic nerve inside the carotid sheath
d. lies superficial to the sternocleidomastoid muscle
e. joins with the subclavian vein to form the brachiocephalic vein.

Question 7

The laryngeal mask airway (LMA):

a. provides no protection against aspiration
b. is particularly easy to use in children
c. is often a suitable alternative to tracheal intubation during CPR
d. is ineffective with capnography
e. requires less cervical spine movement than tracheal intubation during insertion.

Question 8

Pacing:

a. should only be attempted if the patient is refractory to atropine
b. if delivered through percutaneous pads, is painful for an awake patient
c. if performed as fist pacing, should be delivered at a rate of 80–90/min
d. may be effective for an asystolic cardiac arrest
e. may be performed in an emergency by a transcutaneous wire inserted via a central venous catheter into the left ventricle.

Question 9

Fibrinolytic therapy:

a. should not be used routinely in cardiac arrest
b. ongoing CPR is a contraindication to thrombolytic administration
c. is indicated when cardiac arrest is thought to result from a suspected or proven pulmonary embolus
d. with tenecteplase is given as a 500–600 µg/kg IV bolus
e. when administered, requires at least 30 min of further CPR to disrupt any embolus.

Question 10

Open-chest CPR:

a. produces better coronary blood flow than external chest compression
b. may be indicated for traumatic cardiac arrest
c. may be indicated in patients post-cardiac surgery
d. may be indicated in acute pulmonary embolus
e. may be indicated in electromechanical dissociation.

Question 11

The nasopharyngeal airway:

a. should be sized by assessing the diameter of the patient's little finger
b. is relatively contraindicated in patients with a head injury
c. size refers to the external diameter
d. size 8–9 mm is suitable for most adults
e. Causes nasopharyngeal trauma in 30% cases.

Question 12

Adenosine:

a. is indicated for supraventricular tachycardias with re-entrant circuits that include the atrioventricular (AV) node
b. blocks transmission through the AV node
c. may cause prolonged bradycardia
d. is contraindicated in patients with asthma
e. is contraindicated in patients with ischaemic heart disease.

Question 13

In the treatment of anaphylaxis:

a. adrenaline IV is preferable to the IM route if a cannula is in place
b. the standard adult dose of IM adrenaline is 500 µg
c. titrate O_2 to give saturations of 94–98%
d. give children fluid challenges of 10 ml/kg if hypotensive
e. give adults fluid challenges of 500–1000 ml.

Question 14

In the treatment of cardiac arrest caused by asthma:

a. a tracheal tube inserted early in the arrest will facilitate effective airway management
b. manual ventilation should aim to deliver the same respiratory rate and volume as used in standard cardiac arrest management
c. a period of disconnection from the ventilator may reduce gas trapping
d. bilateral chest drains should be inserted to exclude bilateral tension pneumothoraces
e. standard defibrillation energy protocols are indicated.

Question 15

With regard to resuscitation fluids:

a. 0.9% saline is a hypertonic solution
b. Hartmann's solution is an example of a colloid
c. normal saline may cause a metabolic acidosis if given in large volumes
d. Gelofusine and Haemaccel are examples of colloids
e. 5% dextrose is particularly suitable for volume expansion in cardiac arrest.

Question 16

The QT interval:

a. is measured from the start of the QRS complex to the start of the T wave
b. may vary between different leads of the same ECG
c. lengthens as heart rate increases
d. is lengthened by hyperkalaemia and digoxin treatment
e. is lengthened by hypokalaemia and hypothermia.

Question 17

With regard to manual biphasic defibrillator energy levels:

a. 150 J is acceptable as a first shock energy level
b. 200 J is acceptable as a first shock energy level
c. following an initial shock of 150 J, a further 150 J is acceptable as a second shock energy level
d. in a patient who has been shocked back into a perfusing rhythm but who subsequently refibrillates, a shock of 360 J should be administered
e. obese patients may require greater energy levels for successful defibrillation.

Question 18

Thrombophlebitis may be caused by IV administered:

a. amiodarone
b. 50% dextrose
c. hypertonic saline
d. adrenaline
e. atropine.

Question 19

Heliox:

a. comprises 79% helium and 21% O_2
b. is supplied in a brown cylinder
c. reduces work of breathing by increasing the tendency to laminar flow
d. reduces work of breathing by reducing resistance in turbulent flow
e. may assist ventilation in patients with acute severe asthma.

Question 20

With regard to defibrillation safety:

a. supplementary O_2 should be turned off during defibrillation
b. a ventilation bag should be disconnected from the tracheal tube or supraglottic airway and moved at least 1 m away from the patient's chest
c. self-adhesive pads or paddles placed on a hairy chest may risk sparking or arcing in defibrillation, with a resulting fire or explosion
d. a hairy chest must always be shaved before defibrillation
e. electrode gel paste should only be used for paddles if defibrillation gel pads are unavailable.

Photograph questions

Question 1

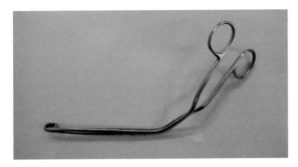

a. What is this implement?
b. What is its function?

Question 2

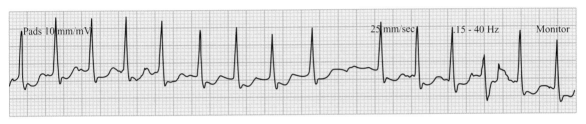

a. What arrhythmia is shown on the ECG trace above?
b. Which arrhythmias can be treated using defibrillation?

Question 3

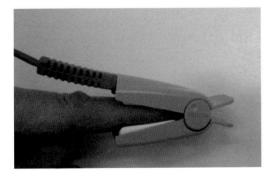

a. What is this device?
b. What are the limitations of this device for measuring respiratory insufficiency?
c. When might a pulse oximeter over-read?

Question 4

Label the heart chambers and great vessels marked A–G in the diagram

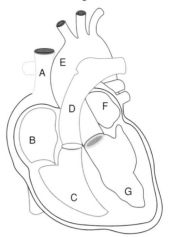

c. What is the risk of a 'blind' shock in these patients?

Question 5

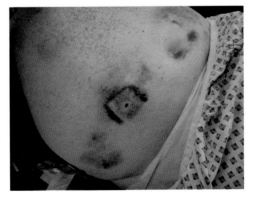

a. What is the cause of bruising on this patient's abdomen?
b. What is this patient's likely clotting status as measured by the activated partial thromboplastin time ratio (APTR)?
c. What is this patient's likely clotting status as measured by the international normalized ratio (INR)?

Diagnostic questions

Question 1

A child presents in the emergency department with the following rhythm:

a. What is this arrhythmia and what percentage of children present with this as the initial rhythm?
b. What are the common causes of this arrhythmia?
c. What is the optimal treatment for this 10 kg child?

Question 2

Complete the following table, indicating drug compatibility (√) or incompatibility (×).

	Water for injection	0.9% Saline	5% Dextrose	Hartmann's solution
Adrenaline				
Atropine				
Amiodarone				
Calcium chloride				

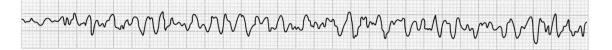

Question 3

This patient presents in a state of haemodynamic collapse.

a. What is the original arrhythmia shown on the ECG below?
b. What is the subsequent rhythm?
c. What drug may have been given to induce this change?

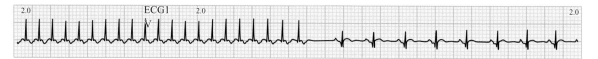

Question 4

The following blood results are measured in an adult with acute severe asthma who has received a magnesium infusion:

Na^+	139 mmol/l
K^+	4.5 mmol/l
Mg^{2+}	9.7 mmol/l
Ca^{2+}	1.1 mmol/l

a. Comment on the magnesium levels.
b. What likely side effects could be expected?
c. What are the treatment options for this condition?

Question 5

This is a posterior–anterior CXR taken in a patient with breathlessness and hypotension following an acute myocardial infarct.

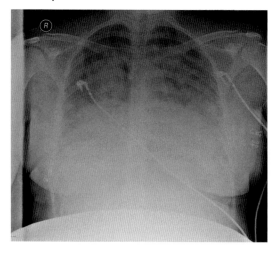

a. What is the likely cause of the breathlessness?
b. What conditions may cause this?

Short answer questions

Question 1

Discuss the management of a patient who has suffered a cardiac arrest caused by accidental electrocution.

Question 2

Discuss the changes in arterial CO_2 ($Paco_2$) in a patient with acute severe asthma as it progresses to life-threatening asthma.

Question 3

What is an Allen's test?

a. Why is it done?
b. How is it performed?

Question 4

A patient who suffers a cardiac arrest has been taking the following drugs:

a. aspirin
b. ramipril
c. steroids.

How may these affect the resuscitation efforts?

Question 5

Draw the algorithm for the treatment of paediatric choking.

MCQ answers

Answer 1

a. **True.**
b. **False.** Should be considered for cardiac arrest associated with hyperkalaemia.
c. **False.** Shifts the O_2 dissociation curve to the left, decreasing O_2 delivery to tissues.
d. **True.**
e. **True.**

Answer 2

a. **False.** Is defined as a core temperature $\geq 37.6°C$.
b. **True.**
c. **False.** Is usually caused by an inflammatory response.
d. **False.** Paracetamol may limit, but does not abolish, pyrexia.
e. **True.**

Answer 3

a. **False.**
b. **True.** May worsen bronchospasm.
c. **False.**
d. **True.** May worsen myocardial function.
e. **True.** May worsen myocardial function.

Answer 4

a. **True.**
b. **False.** Indicates oesophageal placement when the syringe plunger cannot be withdrawn or the bulb will not reinflate.
c. **True.** In these patients, the trachea may collapse when aspiration is attempted.
d. **True.** In these patients, the trachea may collapse when aspiration is attempted.
e. **True.** In these patients, the trachea may collapse when aspiration is attempted.

Answer 5

a. **False.** A dose of 300 mg is recommended.
b. **False.** The risks of a single dose are minimal.
c. **True.**
d. **False.**
e. **True.**

Answer 6

a. **False.** Lies lateral to the carotid artery.
b. **True.**
c. **False.** Runs with the vagus nerve inside the carotid sheath.
d. **False.** Lies deep to the sternocleidomastoid muscle.
e. **True.**

Answer 7

a. **False.** The LMA provides some degree of protection from aspiration.
b. **False.** The LMA tends to be unstable and is associated with more complications than in adults.
c. **True.**
d. **False.** Capnography can be used with all supraglottic airway devices.
e. **True.**

Answer 8

a. **True.**
b. **True.** The patient may require sedation and analgesia.
c. **False.** Should be delivered at a rate of 50–70/min.
d. **False.** Pacing is ineffective in asystolic arrests.
e. **False.** Central venous access allows the wire to be placed in the right ventricle.

Answer 9

a. **True.** The Thrombolysis in Cardiac Arrest (TROICA) trial (Boettiger B *et al. N Engl J Med*, 2008;359:2651–2662) demonstrated no survival benefit for the routine administration of thrombolytics (tenecteplase) during cardiac arrest.
b. **False.**
c. **True.**
d. **True.**
e. **False.** 60–90 min CPR is recommended.

Answer 10

a. **True.**
b. **True.**
c. **True.**
d. **False.**
e. **False.**

Answer 11

a. **False.** This method has been shown to be inaccurate.
b. **True.** Because of risks of cranial injury in patients with a base of skull fracture.
c. **False.** Size refers to internal diameter.
d. **False.** Size 6–7 mm is suitable for most adults.
e. **True.**

Answer 12

a. **True.**
b. **True.**
c. **False.** Adenosine has a very short half-life, with an action of no more than 30 s.
d. **True.**
e. **False.**

Answer 13

a. **False.** The IV route carries considerable risks and should only be used by those with experience of giving IV adrenaline as part of their normal clinical practice (e.g. intensivists, anaesthetists, emergency physicians, etc.).
b. **False.**
c. **False.** Initially, give the highest concentration of O_2 possible using a mask with an O_2 reservoir. Oxygen saturations can be titrated once the patient is stable.
d. **False.** Children should be given 30 ml/kg fluid boluses.
e. **True.**

(See Soar J *et al. Resuscitation*, 2010;81:1400–1433.)

Answer 14

a. **True.** Because airway pressures are much higher in asthmatic patients, bag-valve-mask risks greater gastric insufflation with subsequent diaphragmatic splinting and further hypoventilation.
b. **True.** To deliver 8–10 breaths/min with sufficient tidal volume to observe the chest rising.
c. **True.** Although there is limited evidence for the effectiveness of this manoeuvre.
d. **False.** Although there should be a high index of suspicioun for this pathology.
e. **True.** However, because hyperinflation increases transthoracic impedance, higher energy levels may be considered, although there is no evidence that this increases shock success.

(See Soar J *et al. Resuscitation*, 2010;81:1400–1433.)

Answer 15

a. **False.** 0.9% is a physiologically balanced solution (normal saline).
b. **False.** Hartmann's solution is a crystalloid.
c. **True.**
d. **True.**
e. **False.** Dextrose is redistributed out of the intravascular space rapidly so is poor at maintaining volume expansion. It may also cause hyperglycaemia, which worsens neurological recovery of an ischaemic brain.

Answer 16

a. **False.** Is measured from the start of the QRS complex to the end of the T wave.
b. **True.** This may partly reflect variation in amplitude and direction of the T wave.
c. **False.** The QT interval shortens as the heart rate increases.
d. **False.** The QT interval is shortened by hyperkalaemia and digoxin treatment.
e. **True.**

Answer 17

a. **True.**
b. **True.**
c. **True.** When using a fixed energy protocol.
d. **False.** The patient should be defibrillated using the energy level that last cardioverted them successfully.
e. **False.** Biphasic defibrillators measure transthoracic impedance prior to shock delivery and automatically increase energy output as appropriate. There is no evidence that obese patients require higher energy levels to maintain shock efficacy.

Answer 18

a. **True.**
b. **True.**
c. **True.**
d. **False.**
e. **False.**

Answer 19

a. **True.**
b. **False.** Is supplied in a white cylinder with white/brown shoulders. Brown cylinders are 100% helium.
c. **True.**
d. **True.**
e. **True.**

Answer 20

a. **False.** The O_2 mask/nasal cannulae should be placed at least 1 m away from the patient's chest.
b. **False.** The ventilation bag can be left connected. No increase in O_2 concentrations over the patient's chest have been documented, even with flow rates of 15 l/min.
c. **True.**
d. **False.** Shave the chest over the electrode sites if time permits. In hairy patients, biaxillary electrode placement may be quicker than shaving the chest.
e. **False.** Electrode gel paste may smear across the chest and risk causing a short circuit between paddles. Its use is not recommended.

Photograph answers

Answer 1

a. McGill forceps.
b. For handling structures in the laryngopharynx, for example manual insertion of nasogastric tube or removal of a foreign body.

Answer 2

a. This ECG trace shows a patient in atrial fibrillation with marks showing that the defibrillator is synchronized with the QRS complexes. Synchronization ensures that the DC electrical discharge is synchronized with the R wave of the QRS complex, thus avoiding the shock being inadvertently delivered on the T wave, which may induce VF.
b. The following arrhythmias require synchronized cardioversion:
   - atrial fibrillation
   - atrial flutter
   - AV node re-entrant tachycardia (re-entrant supraventricular tachycardia)
   - ventricular tachycardia.
c. Synchronization aims to avoid energy delivery near the apex of the T wave of the ECG, which coincides with a vulnerable period for induction of VF. 'Blind' defibrillation carries a 5% risk of inducing VF.

Answer 3

a. Pulse oximeter.
b. Although pulse oximetry will measure the O_2 saturation of capillary/arterial blood, this does not correlate with CO_2 elimination or minute volume. Patients, particularly those receiving supplementary O_2, may maintain relatively normal O_2 saturation at very low respiratory rates and low minute volumes. Pulse oximetry measures the adequacy of oxygenation, which is not a measure of the adequacy of ventilation (Davidson JAH, Hosie HE. *BMJ*, 1993;307:372–373).
c. A high level of methaemoglobin will cause the pulse oximeter to read approximately 85%, even if O_2 saturations are lower than this value.

Answer 4

Heart structures:

A: superior vena cava
B: right atrium
C: right ventricle
D: pulmonary artery
E: aorta
F: left atrium
G: left ventricle.

Answer 5

a. Subcutaneous heparin injections, given as prophylaxis for deep vein thrombosis.
b. The APTR is usually unaffected.
c. The INR is usually unaffected.

Diagnostic answers

Answer 1

a. This rhythm strip shows VF. In paediatric cardiac arrest, VF has been documented as the primary arrhythmia in 3.8% cases (asystole in 78.9%, pulseless electrical activity in 13.5%) (Kuisma M *et al. Resuscitation*, 1995;30:141–150).

b. Common causes of VF in children include:
   - congenital heart disease
   - hyperkalaemia
   - hypothermia
   - tricyclic overdose.

c. Appropriate treatment is immediate defibrillation. For both monophasic and biphasic waveforms, the recommended energy level is 4 J/kg, rounded up to the nearest selectable energy level on the defibrillator. Therefore, for a 10 kg child, 40 J would be appropriate. In most manual defibrillators, 50 J would be the nearest appropriate energy level that could be selected.

Answer 2

	Water for injection	0.9% Saline	5% Dextrose	Hartmann's solution
Adrenaline	✓	✓	✓	✓
Atropine	✓	✓	✓	✓
Amiodarone	✓	✓	✓	✓
Calcium chloride	✓		✓	✓

Campbell E, et al. Am J Hosp Pharm. 1986;43:917–921. http://www.resus.org.uk/pages/faqals.htm (See Q3)

Answer 3

a. Supraventricular tachycardia.
b. Sinus rhythm.
c. Adenosine is usually the drug of choice to treat supraventricular tachycardia. (Verapamil may be an alternative in patients without myocardial or valvular heart disease.) This ECG shows the effect of 6 mg IV adenosine, which has terminated the supraventricular tachycardia.

Answer 4

a. Magnesium may be of benefit in patients with acute severe asthma where it has bronchodilator properties. The recommended dose is 2 g magnesium sulphate given as an IV infusion over 10–20 min. The normal magnesium range is 0.8–1.2 mmol/l. A magnesium level of 9.7 mmol/l is significantly elevated (and not likely to occur with 2 g magnesium sulphate).

b. Side effects of hypermagnesaemia include nausea and vomiting, generalized weakness, hypotension, hypocalcaemia and arrhythmias, progressing to asystole. The clinical effects relate to serum concentration (mmol/l):
   - >4.0: hyporeflexia
   - >5.0: prolonged atrioventricular conduction
   - >10.0: complete heart block
   - >12.0: cardiac arrest.

c. Treatment options:
   - IV calcium antagonizes the cardiac and neuromuscular actions of magnesium and may provide acute protection from the arrhythmogenic effects of hypermagnesaemia; this patient has borderline hypocalcaemia and IV calcium may be of particular benefit
   - IV loop diuretics (e.g. furosemide) increase magnesium excretion
   - renal dialysis may be necessary in severe cases, particularly with established renal failure where diuretics are of limited benefit.

Answer 5

a. This CXR shows fulminant pulmonary oedema caused by left ventricular failure, as characterized by:
   - **interstitial oedema**: characteristic bats wing pattern
   - **upper lobe blood diversion**: with more prominent upper lobe vessels
   - **pleural effusions**: loss of the costophrenic angle
   - fluid in fissures
   - **Kerly B (septal) lines**: seen at the lung bases, usually no more than 1 mm thick and 1 cm long, perpendicular to the pleural surface (not visible on this CXR).

b. Pulmonary oedema may be cardiogenic or non-cardiogenic in origin (NB: patchy alveolar infiltrates with air bronchograms are more indicative of non-cardiogenic pulmonary oedema).

   Cardiogenic causes include:
   - heart failure
   - coronary artery disease with left ventricular failure

- cardiac arrhythmias
- fluid overload, e.g. renal failure
- cardiomyopathy
- valvular lesions
  - mitral regurgitation
  - mitral stenosis
  - aortic stenosis
  - aortic regurgitation
- myocarditis and infectious endocarditis.

Non-cardiogenic causes include:

- acute respiratory distress syndrome (ARDS)
- high-altitude pulmonary oedema (>3000 m ($>10\,000$ ft))

- heroin or methadone overdose
- aspirin overdose
- eclampsia in pregnancy
- smoke inhalation
- head trauma (neurogenic pulmonary oedema)
- septic shock
- hypovolaemic shock
- re-expansion pulmonary oedema
- disseminated intravascular coagulopathy (DIC)
- near-drowning
- aspiration.

Short answers

Answer 1

Electrical injury causes 1 death per 200 000 people each year (Soar J *et al. Resuscitation*, 2010;81:1400–1433). Most electrical injuries in adults occur in the workplace, whereas children are most commonly injured at home. Lightning strikes cause 1000 deaths each year. Cardiac arrest from electric shock injuries is usually secondary to:

- respiratory arrest caused by paralysis of the respiratory centre or the respiratory muscles
- cardiac arrhythmias (VF) if the current traverses the myocardium during the vulnerable period (analogous to an R-on-T phenomenon); high-voltage AC current is particularly likely to induce VF.

Standard BLS and ALS should be commenced without delay. In addition:

- early tracheal intubation may be needed before facial burns cause soft tissue swelling, creating a difficult airway
- consider head and spine trauma; immobilize the spine as appropriate
- muscular paralysis, may take several hours to resolve and necessitate ventilatory support
- remove smouldering clothes to prevent further thermal injury
- vigorous fluid therapy is required if there is significant tissue destruction
- early surgical assessment is vital as small electrical entry/exit points may mask extensive soft tissue damage
- exclude traumatic injuries caused by tetanic muscular contraction or by the person being thrown.

Answer 2

In the early stages of acute asthma, hyperventilation causes a drop in Pa_{CO_2} to below normal levels (~4.6 kPa). As the asthma worsens, hyperventilation slows as the patient tires and the Pa_{CO_2} levels will rise to normal. As the asthma progresses and becomes severe, hypoventilation occurs as the patient becomes exhausted and Pa_{CO_2} is likely to rise above 8.0 kPa prior to respiratory arrest.

Answer 3

The Allen's test evaluates collateral circulation to the hand by assessing the patency of both the radial and ulnar arteries. The test aims to ensure that the ulnar artery is able to supply sufficient flow to the hand if the radial artery is occluded.

a. It is usually performed prior to radial artery cannulation or arterial blood gas sampling.
b. (i) The arm is elevated and blood allowed to drain from the hand
   (ii) Pressure is applied over both the ulnar and the radial arteries, of sufficient force to occlude them
   (iii) The arm is lowered and the hand should remain blanched
   (iv) Pressure over the ulnar artery is released and colour should return within 10 s if ulnar blood flow is sufficient.

If colour returns to the hand on release of ulnar artery pressure, it is safe to cannulate the radial artery. If colour does not return or returns slowly, the test is considered negative and the radial artery should not therefore be cannulated.

In practice however, the test is not used routinely. Allen's test has a poor sensitivity and specificity for complications following radial artery cannulation, and the available evidence does not support its routine use prior to radial artery puncture. It is prudent, however, that all patients should have regular clinical observation of their hand and finger blood supply following arterial puncture or cannulation.

Answer 4

a. Aspirin irreversibly inhibits the cyclooxygenase enzyme, which is required for prostaglandin and thromboxane synthesis. Aspirin blocks the formation of thromboxane A_2 in platelets, resulting in inhibition of platelet aggregation. Normal platelet function returns approximately 5 days after cessation of aspirin therapy as new platelets enter the circulation. Patients taking aspirin may be more prone to bleeding, particularly from invasive procedures.
b. Ramipril is an ACE inhibitor. This class of drug inhibits the conversion of angiotensin I to angiotensin II, the latter causing arteriolar vasoconstriction and maintenance of vascular tone. Patients taking ACE inhibitors generally have lower blood pressure than normal. While blood pressure may be in the normal range, ACE inhibitors may contribute significantly to any

hypotension during cardiovascular collapse. In patients taking ACE inhibitors, consideration should be given to the use of vasoconstrictor drugs such as noradrenaline or phenylephrine to reverse hypotension caused by these drugs.

c. Corticosteroids are produced in the adrenal cortex and are involved in a wide range of physiological systems, including the stress response, immune response and regulation of inflammation. Patients taking steroids long term have a downregulation of their own endogenous steroid-producing pathways. Sudden cessation of exogenous steroid therapy can, therefore, lead to acute side effects caused by a relative lack of steroid. These side effects include hypotension, hypoglycaemia, hyperkalaemia, hypercalcaemia and convulsions. Patients taking oral steroids prior to their cardiac arrest are likely to require steroid supplementation in the immediate post-arrest phase to maintain normal physiological functioning.

Answer 5

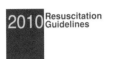

Resuscitation Council (UK)

Paediatric Choking Treatment Algorithm

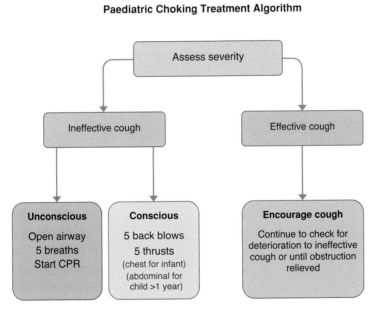

Reproduced with permission from the Resuscitation Council (UK).

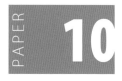

Multiple choice questions

Question 1

With regard to automatic internal cardioverter devices (AICD):

a. a ring magnet placed over the device will trigger defibrillation
b. triggering may occur if the sensing electrode is fractured
c. external defibrillation is contraindicated if an AICD is firing
d. triggering may occur with external chest compression
e. may cause electrical shocks to the rescuer.

Question 2

Therapeutic hypothermia for patients who remain comatose following return of spontaneous circulation:

a. can be induced by iced saline given as an IV bolus of 10 ml/kg
b. is contraindicated following paediatric cardiac arrest
c. may cause an increase in diuresis
d. is associated with an increased risk of pneumonia
e. should be induced for 48 h.

Question 3

The following are associated with increased risk of arrhythmias:

a. hyponatraemia
b. hypokalaemia
c. hypothyroidism
d. hyopcalcaemia
e. hypoglycaemia.

Question 4

With regard to drowning:

a. when unwitnessed, all drowning victims should be treated with cervical spine immobilization until the cervical spine can be cleared

b. compression-only CPR is relatively contraindicated
c. drying a wet patient with a towel does not allow safe defibrillation using self-adhesive pads
d. if core temperature is below 30°C, defibrillation should be limited to no more than three attempts
e. IV fluids may be indicated to correct hypovolaemia caused by the hydrostatic pressure of the water on the body.

Question 5

The sinoatrial (SA) node of the heart:

a. is located in the right atrium of the heart, close to the superior vena cava
b. consists of non-contractile myocytes
c. usually receives blood from the left coronary artery, meaning that a myocardial infarction occluding this artery may cause ischaemia in the SA node
d. is richly innervated by parasympathetic nervous system fibres from the vagus nerve
e. is richly innervated by sympathetic nervous system fibres.

Question 6

Atrial flutter:

a. is a risk factor for stroke
b. is caused by a re-entrant rhythm, typically originating from the left atrium and most often involving a left atrial circuit
c. when untreated, generally results in every second atrial flutter beat conducted to the atrioventricular node, resulting in a heart rate of about 150 beats/min
d. usually progresses to atrial fibrillation
e. is more sensitive to electrical cardioversion than atrial fibrillation, and usually requires a lower energy shock.

Question 7

Common causes of VF cardiac arrest in children include:

a. hypokalaemia
b. hypothermia
c. congenital heart disease
d. Calpol (paracetamol) overdose
e. hypoxaemia.

Question 8

Heat stroke:

a. is defined as a core temperature $>40.6°C$, accompanied by mental state change and organ dysfunction
b. is relatively common in the elderly
c. risk factors include dehydration, obesity and alcohol
d. mortality ranges from 10 to 50%
e. therapeutic hypothermia following return of spontaneous circulation is not indicated in heat stroke patients.

Question 9

Verapamil:

a. is a calcium channel agonist
b. slows conduction in the atrioventricular node
c. is indicated for supraventricular tachycardias unresponsive to vagal manoeuvres or adenosine
d. is particularly effective for ventricular tachycardia
e. is given as slow 2.5–5 mg IV bolus.

Question 10

End-tidal CO_2 measurements are affected by:

a. the minute ventilation delivered during resuscitation
b. lung disease that increases anatomic dead space
c. presence of right-to-left shunting
d. administration of adrenaline
e. percentage O_2 delivered by the ventilation circuit.

Question 11

The rate of fluid flow in a cannula:

a. is inversely proportional to its length
b. is proportional to the square of the cannula radius
c. is slowed by turbulent flow
d. is proportional to fluid viscosity
e. is determined by the pressure in the vein in which the cannula sits.

Question 12

Lightning injuries:

a. commonly cause VF
b. may cause prolonged respiratory arrest
c. rarely cause direct cardiac arrest
d. commonly cause severe deep burns
e. typically involve 300 000 V delivered over 5–10 ms.

Question 13

Digoxin:

a. is a cardiac glycoside extracted from the foxglove plant, *Digitalis lanata*
b. decreases vagal tone
c. prolongs atrioventricular node refractory period
d. decreases the PR interval
e. plasma levels are increased in patients taking amiodarone.

Question 14

Therapeutic hypothermia may cause:

a. hyperphosphataemia
b. hyperkalaemia
c. hypermagnesaemia
d. hypocalcaemia
e. hyponatraemia.

Question 15

With regard to heart block:

a. first-degree heart block may be a normal variant in 1% of young adults
b. in second-degree heart block, a P wave is blocked from initiating a QRS complex
c. type 1 (Wenckebach) second-degree heart block is considered more benign than type 2 second-degree heart block
d. third-degree is also known as complete heart block
e. third-degree heart block may be associated with an escape rhythm.

Question 16

With regard to poisoning:

a. gastric lavage is only of benefit if performed within 1 h of the ingestion of the poison
b. emetics (e.g. ipecacuanha) are only of benefit if given within 1 h of the ingestion of the poison
c. haemodialysis may be of benefit for ethylene glycol (antifreeze) poisoning
d. haemodialysis may be of benefit for lithium poisoning
e. charcoal haemoperfusion may be of benefit for paracetamol poisoning.

Question 17

In the treatment of supraventricular tachycardia:

a. adenosine is the first-line treatment
b. carotid sinus massage may act by decreasing sympathetic tone
c. carotid sinus massage may cause a transient ischaemic attack or stroke
d. a Valsalva manoeuvre (forced expiration against a closed glottis) is a suitable alternative to carotid sinus massage
e. an ECG should be performed after each manoeuvre to assess any change in rhythm.

Question 18

The oropharyngeal airway:

a. was designed by Arthur Guedel
b. is sized by measuring the distance from the corner of the patient's mouth to the angle of the mandible
c. is inserted inverted in adults
d. is inserted inverted in children
e. should be inverted as it is removed from an adult's airway.

Question 19

Biphasic waveforms:

a. consist of two peaks of current delivered in quick succession
b. are less influenced by transthoracic impedance than the older monophasic waveforms
c. should be delivered using at least 100 J for the initial shock
d. effectiveness is determined by the polarity of the electrodes: the direction of current flow from sternal to apical pad
e. should be delivered at the same energy level for children as monophasic defibrillation.

Question 20

With regard to tricyclic antidepressant overdose:

a. common tricyclic antidepressants include citalopram, fluoxetine and sertraline.
b. overdose is usually accidental
c. most life-threatening problems occur within the first 2 h after ingestion
d. sodium bicarbonate may be of benefit during resuscitation attempts
e. lipid emulsion (Intralipid) may be of benefit during resuscitation attempts.

Photograph questions

Question 1

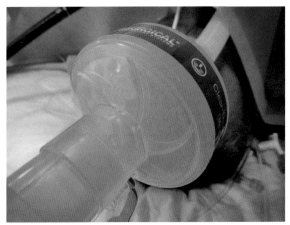

a. What is this device?
b. What is its function?

Question 2

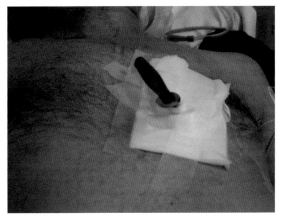

a. What are the cardiac chambers commonly injured in penetrating injuries such as this?
b. The patient is hypotensive with distended neck veins. What is the likely pathology?
c. What treatment would you consider while waiting for the cardiac surgeons to arrive?

Question 3

Chain of survival

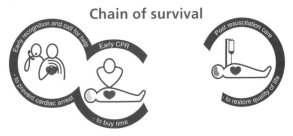

a. What is the missing link in this chain of survival?
b. What increase in mortality per minute results from failure to implement this missing link?
c. Where is the nearest device to allow you to implement this missing link?

Question 4

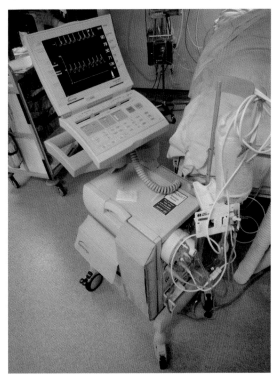

a. What is this device?
b. Draw an arterial pressure waveform seen in a patient when this device is in use.

Question 5

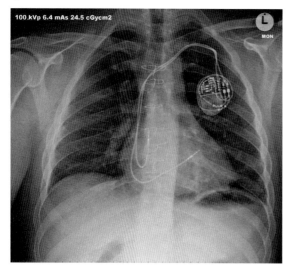

a. What implanted device is shown in this CXR?
b. Where is it anatomically positioned?
c. What additional procedure has been undertaken in this patient?

Diagnostic questions

Question 1

Occupational therapy test you for immunity to hepatitis B following a needlestick injury acquired during the resuscitation of a patient. Your serology results show the following:

- HBsAg (hepatitis B surface antigen): negative
- Anti-HBc (hepatitis B core antibody): negative
- Anti-HBs (hepatitis B surface antibody): positive.
  a. Do these results show that you are immune to hepatitis B?
  b. How does serology differ in individuals with immunity resulting from a previous hepatits B infection rather than the vaccination?

Question 2

This is a transthoracic echo of a patient who presents to the emergency department with decompensated heart failure.

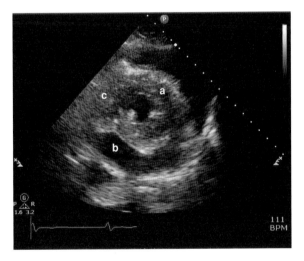

a. What view is shown?
b. Name the structures (a), (b) and (c).

Question 3

A patient is brought to the emergency department having been rescued from a house fire. Their arterial blood gas on air show a carboxyhaemoglobin (HbCO) level of 35%.

a. How significant is this level?
b. Is any specific treatment required?

Question 4

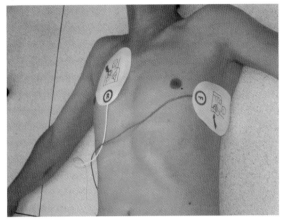

a. Are these self-adhesive pads placed correctly?
b. What is the difference in electrode placement for attempted defibrillation of atrial fibrillation and VF?
c. What are the recommendations for orientation of the apical electrode?

Question 5

A patient presents with a serum potassium of 7.7 mmol/l. What are the possible causes of hyperkalaemia?

Short answer questions

Question 1

When may thrombolysis be indicated during a cardiac arrest?

Question 2

Write short notes on the post-cardiac arrest syndrome.

Question 3

A young adult is admitted in cardiac arrest who has been taking cocaine. Why may cocaine cause a cardiac arrest? What modifications or additions to the standard ALS protocol may be necessary during the attempt to resuscitate him?

Question 4

How can correct positioning of an IO needle be verified?

Question 5

Write short notes on pulmonary aspiration during cardiac arrest.

MCQ answers

Answer 1

a. **False.** A magnet placed over the device will deactivate the defibrillation function.
b. **True.**
c. **False.** Internal defibrillator discharge will only continue to occur if a patient remains in a shockable rhythm. In these circumstances, external defibrillation is indicated.
d. **False.**
e. **True.** Cases of electrical shocks being felt by the rescuer have been reported.

Answer 2

a. **False.** Saline should be administered at 30 ml/kg.
b. **False.** Cooling is not contraindicated, although evidence for its efficacy only comes from adult studies.
c. **True.**
d. **True.**
e. **False.** Current guidelines are that therapeutic hypothermia should be induced for 12–24 h.

Answer 3

a. **False.**
b. **True.**
c. **False.** Although bradycardia is common.
d. **False.**
e. **False.**

Answer 4

a. **False.** Cervical spine injury is rare (<0.5%) and immobilization is not indicated unless history or physical signs suggest severe injury.
b. **True.** Most drowning victims have suffered a cardiac arrest caused by hypoxaemia; the ventilation component of BLS is, therefore, vital.
c. **False.** Self-adhesive pads can be used safely if the patient is first dried with a towel.
d. **True.** Drug therapy should also be withheld until core temperature is >30°C.
e. **True.**

Answer 5

a. **True.**
b. **True.**
c. **False.** Usually receives blood from the right coronary artery, meaning that a myocardial infarction occluding this artery may cause ischaemia in the SA node.
d. **True.**
e. **True.**

Answer 6

a. **True.**
b. **False.** Atrial flutter usually arises from the right atrium, and involves a right atrial circuit.
c. **True.**
d. **True.**
e. **True.**

Answer 7

a. **False.** Hyperkalaemia
b. **True.** Core generally <28°C.
c. **True.**
d. **True.**
e. **False.** Hypoxaemia generally causes bradycardia, progressing to asystole.

Answer 8

a. **True.**
b. **True.** The elderly are at increased risk for heat-related illness because they have less ability for self-care and declining thermoregulatory mechanisms.
c. **True.** Also cardiovascular disease, skin conditions (psoriasis, eczema), hyperthyroidism and some drugs (anticholinergics, opioids, cocaine, amphetamine, phenothiazines, calcium channel blockers, β-blockers).
d. **True.**
e. **False.** Patients resuscitated from heat stroke-induced cardiac arrest should be cooled as for normal cardiac arrest.

Answer 9

a. **False.** Verapamil is a calcium channel antagonist.
b. **True.**
c. **True.**
d. **False.** Verapamil may cause cardiovascular collapse when given to patients in ventricular tachycardia.
e. **True.**

133

Answer 10

a. **True.** Increasing minute volume decreases end-tidal CO_2 by the same proportion.
b. **True.**
c. **True.** Right-to-left shunting decreases the amount of CO_2 delivered to the pulmonary vascular tree.
d. **True.** Adrenaline (and other systemic vasoconstrictors) transiently decrease end-tidal CO_2.
e. **False.**

Answer 11

The rate of fluid flow in a cannula (ϕ) is given by the Hagen–Pouiselle equation:

$$\phi = \frac{\pi r^4 \Delta P}{8 \eta L}$$

where r is the internal radius of the tube (metres), ΔP the pressure difference between the two ends (pascals), η the dynamic fluid viscosity (pascal-second (Pa s)) and L the total length of the tube.

a. **True.**
b. **False.**
c. **True.**
d. **False.**
e. **True.**

Answer 12

a. **False.** Commonly cause transient asystole from which the heart recovers spontaneously.
b. **True.**
c. **True.** Cardiac arrest is usually secondary to hypoxia from a respiratory arrest.
d. **False.** Most lightning strikes cause superficial burns. Deep burns are rare.
e. **True.**

Answer 13

a. **True.**
b. **False.** Increases vagal tone.
c. **True.**
d. **False.** Increases the PR interval by slowing atrioventricular conduction.
e. **True.** By displacing tissue binding sites and depressing renal digoxin clearance.

Answer 14

a. **False.** Hypophosphataemia.
b. **False.** Hypokalaemia.
c. **False.** Hypomagnesaemia.
d. **True.**
e. **False.**

Answer 15

a. **True.**
b. **True.**
c. **True.**
d. **True.**
e. **True.** Because the impulse is blocked, an accessory pacemaker in the ventricular wall will typically activate the ventricles. This is known as an escape rhythm.

Answer 16

a. **True.**
b. **False.** Emetics have no role in the modern management of poisoning.
c. **True.**
d. **True.**
e. **False.** Charcoal haemoperfusion may be of benefit for intoxication with carbamazepine, phenobarbital, phenytoin or theophylline.

Answer 17

a. **False.** Vagal manoeuvres are the first line treatment.
b. **False.** Carotid sinus massage stimulates baroreceptors, which increase vagal tone.
c. **True.** It should not be performed if a bruit (suggestive of an atheromatous plaque) is audible with a stethoscope.
d. **True.**
e. **False.** An ECG should be performed during each manoeuvre to assess the underlying rhythm as the ventricular response slows.

Answer 18

a. **True.**
b. **False.** Are sized by measuring from the corner of the patient's mouth to the tip of the earlobe.
c. **True.**
d. **False.**
e. **False.**

Answer 19

a. **False.** Biphasic waveforms consist of a positive phase, followed immediately by a negative phase.
b. **True.** Biphasic waveforms are modified by the defibrillator according to the transthoracic impedance and their efficacy is, therefore, unaffected by its variations.
c. **False.** The initial shock should be at least 150 J (although 120 J is acceptable for biphasic rectilinear waveforms).
d. **False.** Biphasic efficacy is not determined by direction of current flow.
e. **True.** Delivery of 4 J/kg is recommended for a child, irrespective of whether the defibrillator is monophasic or biphasic.

Answer 20

a. **False.** Tricyclic antidepressants include amitriptyline, desipramine, imipramine, nortriptyline, doxepin and clomipramine).
b. **False.** Overdose in adults is usually deliberate.
c. **False.** Most life-threatening problems occur within the first 6 h after ingestion.
d. **True.**
e. **True.**

Photograph answers

Answer 1

a. This is a heat and moisture exchange filter. It sits in the respiratory circuit where:
   - it is warmed by expired air, resulting in the subsequent warming of inspired air
   - condensation from expired air on the filter adds moisture to inspired air.

b. It acts as a filter to protect the proximal breathing circuit from microbiological contamination.

Answer 2

a. In stab wounds to the chest, the right ventricle is the most commonly injured cardiac chamber (45% of cases). The left ventricle is injured in 35%, right atrium in 10% and left atrium in 5%.

b. Cardiac tamponade.

c. Needle pericardiocentesis, preferably using transthoracic echocardiography to guide needle placement.

Answer 3

a. Early defibrillation to restart the heart.

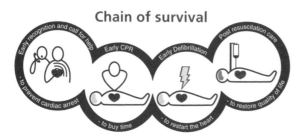

b. Delays to defibrillation without bystander CPR increase mortality at a rate of 7–10% per minute.

c. Automatic external defibrillators (AEDs) are commonly located in areas of high public density such as shopping centres, airports and stations.

Answer 4

a. This is an intra-aortic balloon pump (IABP).

b. The arterial waveform seen when the device is used is shown below.

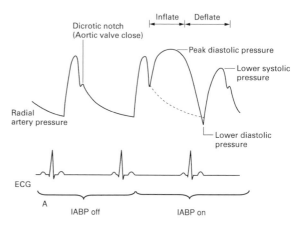

Answer 5

a. Dual chamber pacemaker. (Two leads can be seen: one placed in the right atrium, the other in the right ventricle.)

b. Below the left clavicle to the left of the sternum. It is external to the thoracic cage, usually being buried below the pectoral muscles.

c. Wires can been seen in the midline of the sternum, suggesting that this patient has had a previous sternotomy (which necessitates closure of the divided sternum using wires).

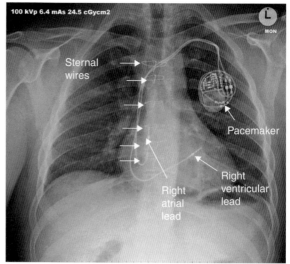

Diagnostic answers

Answer 1

a. Yes. These results suggest a previous hepatitis B vaccination that has resulted in production of anti-HBs. The HBsAg and anti-HBc levels are negative, suggesting no exposure to an actual live virus.

b. In patients exposed to a live virus, anti-HBc (antibodies to the core protein of hepatitis B) will be present (but do not develop following vaccination).

Answer 2

a. Transgastric short axis view.

b. The views are (a) left ventricle, (b) pericardial effusion (probably blood), and (c) thrombus within the pericardial space.

Answer 3

Carbon monoxide has a complex mechanism of action through several pathways, including binding to haemoglobin, myoglobin and mitochondrial cytochrome oxidase. Carbon monoxide is also known to cause brain lipid peroxidation. Toxicity partly arises from the binding of carbon monoxide with haemoglobin to form carboxyhaemoglobin (HbCO), decreasing the O_2-carrying capacity of the blood. Carbon monoxide has a 230 times greater affinity for haemoglobin than O_2; as a result, relatively low levels of carbon monoxide can have a significant impact on O_2-carrying capacity.

Levels of HbCO do not reliably predict clinical symptoms and should only be used as a guide to exposure; treatment of clinical symptoms is of greater priority. Carboxyhaemoglobin blood levels may reach 8–10% in heavy smokers. Symptoms begin as blood levels reach 10–30%. Fatalities have been documented with blood levels of 30–90%.

a. A HbCO level of 35% is significant and suggests prolonged carbon monoxide exposure.

b. Treatment will depend on the symptoms. The immediate priority is to give 100% O_2, which reduces the HbCO half-life from approximately 320 min to 80 min. Significant symptoms such as arrhythmias, seizures, hypotension and pulmonary oedema will need to be treated as appropriate. Hyperbaric O_2 therapy has not been proven to improve long- or short-term outcome.

Answer 4

a. Yes. The right (sternal) electrode is placed to the right of the sternum, below the clavicle. The apical paddle is placed in the left mid-axillary line, approximately level with the V6 ECG electrode or female breast. This position should be clear of any breast tissue. It is important that this electrode is placed sufficiently laterally.

b. There is no difference in recommended electrode position for atrial and ventricular arrhythmias. Acceptable pad positions for all arrhythmias include:

   - placement of each electrode on the lateral chest walls, one on the right and the other on the left side (bi-axillary)
   - one electrode in the standard apical position and the other on the right upper back
   - one electrode anteriorly, over the left precordium, and the other electrode posteriorly to the heart just inferior to the left scapula.

c. There is no evidence that the orientation of the apical pad (cranio-caudal or transverse) influences the success of biphasic defibrillation. When using a biphasic defibrillator, the apical electrode (self-adhesive or paddle) may, therefore, be orientated in either a cranio-caudal or transverse orientation.

Answer 5

Causes of hyperkalaemia include:

- renal failure
- drugs
  - ACE inhibitors
  - angiotensin II receptor antagonists
  - potassium-sparing diuretics
  - non-steroidal anti-inflammatory drugs
  - β-blockers
  - trimethoprim
- tissue breakdown (rhabdomyolysis, tumour lysis, haemolysis)
- metabolic acidosis
- endocrine disorders
- Addison's disease
- hyperkalaemic periodic paralysis
- haemolysis (spuriously high reading).

Short answers

Answer 1

Fibrinolytic therapy should not be used routinely in cardiac arrest. The Thrombolysis in Cardiac Arrest (TROICA) trial (Boettiger B *et al. N Engl J Med*, 2008;359:2651–2662) showed that there was no additional benefit from the use of tenecteplase in the setting of witnessed cardiac arrest of presumed cardiac origin. Fibrinolytic therapy should, however, be considered when cardiac arrest is thought to be caused by proven or suspected acute pulmonary embolus. On-going CPR is not a contraindication to thrombolysis.

Answer 2

The post-cardiac arrest syndrome (Neumar R *et al. Circulation*, 2008;118:2452–2483) is a unique and complex combination of pathophysiological processes, which include:

- brain injury: coma, seizures, cognitive dysfunction, stroke
- myocardial dysfunction: reduced cardiac output, hypotension, dysrrhythmias
- systemic ischaemia/reperfusion response: ongoing tissue hypoxia/ischaemia, pyrexia, hyperglycaemia, multiorgan failure, sepsis
- unresolved pathological process that caused the cardiac arrest.

Clinically, the syndrome is divided into five different stages:

1	20 min	Immediate (return of circulation)
2	20 min to 6–12 h	Early
3	6–12 h to 72 h	Intermediate
4	72 h to discharge	Recovery
5	Discharge onwards	Rehabilitation

Although whole-body ischaemia resulting from the cessation of perfusion during the actual cardiac arrest initially causes global tissue and organ injury, additional damage occurs during and after reperfusion. This later phase of damage is probably related to complex inflammatory pathways, fuelled by free radial oxygen damage.

The severity of these disorders after return of spontaneous circulation is variable and unpredictable, although related broadly to the duration of no-flow time and influenced by the cause of cardiac arrest and the patient's prior state of health. If return of spontaneous circulation is achieved rapidly after onset of cardiac arrest, the post-cardiac arrest syndrome will not occur.

Treatment is aimed at reducing the inflammatory component of this response (through therapeutic hypothermia), optimizing haemodynamic status (inotropes, intra-aortic balloon pump) and optimizing metabolic and acid–base balance.

Answer 3

Cocaine causes massive sympathetic stimulation, resulting in hypertension and tachyarrhythmias. Cardiac arrest may result from myocardial arrhythmias or heart failure. CNS toxicity may result in seizures, cerebral haemorrhage, stroke and cardiorespiratory depression. Cocaine is also a pyrogen, causing an increase in heat production through increased muscular activity and reduced heat loss through global vasoconstriction. Cocaine-induced hyperthermia may cause muscle necrosis and myoglobinuria, with subsequent acidosis and acute renal failure. In managing a patient in cardiac arrest secondary to cocaine overdose, consider the following.

- Drug users may be at greater risk of hepatitis and HIV infection.
- Excessive sympathetic activity may need to be specifically treated. Pure β-blockers should not be used alone because unopposed α-adrenoceptor activity may worsen hypertension. β-blockers may be safely used in conjunction with α-blockers; alternatively, a combined α- and β-blocker (e.g. labetolol) may be used.
- Nitrates may be of benefit if the ECG shows evidence of myocardial ischaemia.
- Consider aortic dissection and intracranial bleeding, both of which are associated with cocaine use.
- Hyperthermia may need specific treatment (active cooling) in the post-resuscitation phase.

Answer 4

Several methods have been described to indicate correct IO needle placement.

- With the initial placement of the device, there is a sudden loss of resistance as the needle passes from the hard outer cortex of the bone to the softer central marrow.
- Once inserted, the needle should stand upright and feel secure with minimal movement.

- Usually small amounts of bone marrow may be aspirated.
- Once the needle is inserted, fluid should be able to be infused through the needle with minimal resistance.
- Surrounding tissues should be regularly assessed for signs of extravasation.

Answer 5

After cardiac arrest, the oesophageal sphincter pressure decreases rapidly from 20 to 5 cmH$_2$O, allowing gastric contents to track back up the oesophagus and enter the trachea. Gastric regurgitation is relatively common at cardiac arrest. It occurs in approximately 30% of out-of-hospital cardiac arrests and, in most of these cases, before the arrival of the ambulance. Pulmonary aspiration after cardiac arrest has been documented in 20% of survivors. The effect of aspiration on achieving return of spontaneous circulation and neurologically intact hospital survival is not known.

Tracheal intubation isolates the trachea and protects it from aspiration, although morbidity from trachea intubation in unskilled hands may offset this benefit. Supraglottic airway devices do appear to afford some degree of protection from aspiration although the incidence of aspiration when using these devices is not documented.

Index

145